Pelvic Prep School

PELVIC PREP
SCHOOL

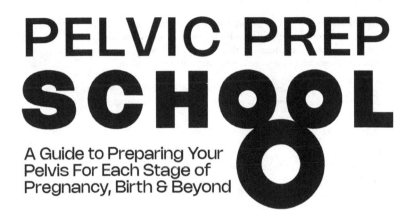

A Guide to Preparing Your
Pelvis For Each Stage of
Pregnancy, Birth & Beyond

DR. SAM DUFLO

PT, DPT, PRPC, RRCA

NEW YORK

LONDON • NASHVILLE • MELBOURNE • VANCOUVER

PELVIC PREP SCHOOL

A Guide to Preparing Your Pelvis for Each Stage of Pregnancy, Birth & Beyond

Published in New York, New York, by Morgan James Publishing. Morgan James is a trademark of Morgan James, LLC. www.MorganJamesPublishing.com

No claim to copyright is made for original U.S. Government Works.

Disclaimer
This book is not intended to be a substitute for medical care or advice from a pelvic physical therapist or physician tailored to your physical needs. You should always undergo an evaluation and seek the advice of your physician or physical therapist prior to engaging in any new physical activity. You should cease activities if you feel symptoms such as shortness of breath, fatigue, physical discomfort, or similar symptoms.

Proudly distributed by Publishers Group West®

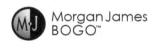

ISBN 9781636982168 paperback
ISBN 9781636982175 ebook
Library of Congress Control Number: 2023937322

Cover Design by:
Alexa Thompson
alexathompsondesign.com

Interior Design by:
Chris Treccani
www.3dogcreative.net

Illustrations by:
Kaysia Grow

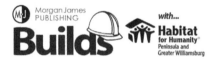

Morgan James is a proud partner of Habitat for Humanity Peninsula and Greater Williamsburg. Partners in building since 2006.

Get involved today! Visit: www.morgan-james-publishing.com/giving-back

For my daughter, my wildfire.
Becoming your mother inspired me to seek answers.
Your magic and spirit led me to who I am today.
–Mama

(Hey Dad, I'm living my dash.)

TABLE OF CONTENTS

ACKNOWLEDGMENTS

First and foremost, I would like to thank my clients: without you, there would be no book. Your stories and self-advocacy have inspired me for over a decade, and for that I could not be more grateful. The encouragement, support and management from my PR Manager, Allison Benson O'Brien, was unmatched, and for that I will be forever thankful. To my publishing team at Morgan James Publishing, thank you for fiercely believing in me and the importance of getting this information out to pregnant people and their partners. Julie Hove Anderson, my photographer, Kaysia Grow, my illustrator, and Jess Gill, my copyeditor: thank you for enduring rounds of edits, lending your expertise and helping to make this manuscript everything I had hoped for. Kelsey H Lucas and Jess Waller: for your input when this was just a seedling. For the Indigo team: I am awestruck every day by your brilliance and perseverance in the field of pelvic health.

Lastly, to my brave, wild and perceptive daughter, my friends, family, loved ones and the circle of women and entrepreneurs that I surround myself with that lift me up and challenge me to be the best version of myself every day: thank you. For my Mom, who gave me the gift of a love for the written word. Dr. Amanda Rich, Dr. Kristen Joyce, and Nicole "T" Andrew: my sisters, supporters, lifelines, and biggest fan club, my love and appreciation for you is indescribable.

It takes a vision AND a village.

Dr. Sam

WELCOME

Hi, friends!

Welcome to Pelvic Prep School: I'm so happy you're here, and I'm sending you the warmest congratulations and well-wishes during this extraordinary time in your life. I believe birth and pregnancy are transformative, empowering, and beautiful. As a pregnant or gestating person, you deserve to feel safe, empowered, and healthy throughout your pregnancy and birth—and I'm here to support you along the journey.

This curated resource includes key information from a pelvic physical therapist's perspective, starting with a better understanding of how your pelvis functions during pregnancy and delivery. You'll learn that you're not destined to pee your pants forever just because you've had a baby. You'll discover that kegels aren't right for everyone, and that any type of pelvic pain needs and deserves to be addressed. I'll walk you through the exercises, stretches, and techniques that are specifically designed to prepare *your* body for birth—with effective tactics to help reduce the risk of tearing during delivery. And along the way, you'll find all of the invaluable tips and suggestions I regularly share with my clients.

The result is a guide that will help you feel empowered and physically capable of the labor and delivery you envision. Regardless of the way your baby is conceived, carried, or brought into this world, I hope that these lessons help you embrace your inner pelvic power and carry you towards a strong and healthy pregnancy, delivery, and postpartum recovery.

Dr. Sam DuFlo, PT, DPTP, PRPC

INTRODUCTION

You shouldn't need to schedule an appointment or scroll aimlessly through questionable content online to understand your pregnant and postpartum body. Pelvic Prep School is designed for the busy pregnant person looking to learn about how their body and their life may change during pregnancy. The pelvis and pelvic floor are a major part of pregnancy, labor, birth, and recovery, and are so often ignored. I'm here to change that!

I'm going to educate you, support you, get you moving, and help you feel better connected to your changing body. And I'm going to start with the most common questions and topics.

As a practitioner, many of the pregnant persons who come to me are looking to continue working or remain physically active, increase their chances of a vaginal birth, learn more about how to avoid tearing, and prepare during pregnancy to best facilitate post-birth recovery. The information in Pelvic Prep School is formulated to help you do just that. I also want to be very clear: all birth, regardless of the method of delivery, is natural. Nurturing a growing body inside yours and bringing that new light into the world is as natural as it gets!

All birth = Natural birth

In the coming pages, you'll become empowered with the tools and knowledge you need to have an informed pregnancy and go into the postpartum phase feeling power over your body. With this guide, you'll:

1. **Become familiar** with the pelvic floor muscles and basic anatomy of the pelvis—you know, the thing housing your baby!
2. **Understand** why these muscles are important for labor and delivery.
3. **Learn** why kegels might not be right for you and how you can prepare for pushing safely and confidently.
4. **Discover** what to safely do during pregnancy to prepare your pelvis for labor, birth and delivery, and beyond.

Just One More Thing Before We Jump In

Rising printing costs prevented me from being able to produce the book in full color and keep it at a practical price point for you. But I much prefer the full color versions of our images and photography as they lend valuable definition to certain details.

So we created a full color guide to go hand-in-hand with the material in this book. Download it for free using the QR code below.

Until you feel you have a deep understanding of the context for each technique and how to execute them, I want you to keep this copy handy for continued learning and step-by-step instructions while using the image guide.

Now without further ado, let's get started.

PART 1:

PREGNANCY & YOUR PELVIS

CHAPTER 1:

Understanding Your Pelvis

Hello, meet your pelvis

The pelvis is the root of your pregnancy: housing the pelvic organs, stabilizing your growing body, and fostering the growth of your baby.

Why understand your pelvis?

The better you understand your own anatomy and what is typical for you, the better you can advocate for yourself during gestation, pregnancy, and birth. From working with numerous new mothers and birthing parents over the years, I've discovered that a lot of pregnant people have major gaps in knowledge of their own bodies. But knowing how your body works is key to understanding how to best support yourself during this time. Learning what's normal for your body can help you identify and further articulate your needs when things don't feel normal to you. Trust your gut (or in this case, your pelvis!)

But First: 7 Things to Know About Your Pelvic Floor

1. **Your pelvic floor is a group of muscles that can be exercised.** In fact, it is three layers of muscles that both contract and relax, and have voluntary and involuntary actions, meaning some things you control (squeeze!) and others you don't.

2. **But kegels can sometimes do more harm than good.** Overuse through excessive or inappropriate contractions can lead to poor lengthening of the muscles for delivery, a painful tailbone, or painful sex.

3. **Peeing your pants after pregnancy is not normal.** Let us repeat: Not. Normal. This is where pelvic physical therapists can help!

4. Pain during sex after pregnancy is also not normal. Common, but not normal.

5. Your vagina won't feel "looser" after pregnancy. Different, maybe.

6. You should see a pelvic floor physical therapist during pregnancy. Not just postpartum.

7. A pelvic floor physical therapist is intimate but not invasive.

Pelvic Organs

If you haven't thought about anatomy since sex-ed in high school, it's time for a mini lesson. The pelvis is designed to provide a safe and protected home for the pelvic organs, such as the uterus, bladder, and rectum, as well as help to stabilize the core and assist the body and legs in propelling the body forward during movement, provide an outlet for birth, and distribute weight throughout.

Here are the key players:

Uterus: For menstruation and the development of the fetus, where the placenta is housed

Bladder: Holding tank for urine, which sits under the front of the uterus

Urethra: Tube connecting the bladder that lets out your urine

Rectum: Holding tank for poop

Anus: Sphincter that lets out your poop

Clitoris: Sexual pleasure center that both houses nerve endings externally and wraps around internally

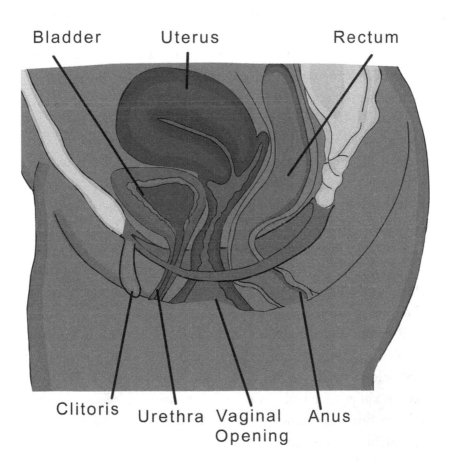

Bladder   Uterus   Rectum

Clitoris   Urethra   Vaginal Opening   Anus

Let's Dive Deeper

Now that we've gotten the basics out of the way, let's talk about how these anatomic features play a role throughout your pregnancy.

Uterus: The uterus is a hollow, muscular organ that sits between the rectum and the bladder in the pelvis. The uterus connects to the uterine tubules, which carry the egg from the ovary to the uterus for implantation once fertilized. The lining of the uterus—the endometrium—grows and thickens during parts of the menstrual cycle to provide a home for the fertilized egg to implant. If there is no fertilized egg, the lining sheds (your period.) The uterus is essential for fertility, menstruation, and pregnancy. It grows in tandem with the growing baby and placenta, experiences strong contractions during birthing, then heals over time to resume its normal size and location postpartum.

Bladder: The bladder sits in front of and slightly below the front of the uterus and holds urine. As your baby grows and your uterus enlarges, there is more pressure on the bladder and less room for its expansion (read: it fills up faster.) This is what causes the increase in the number of times you feel like you have to urinate during pregnancy.

Urethra: This tube connects the bladder to the exit in front of the vagina. The urethra tube holds two sphincters (muscular structures that can contract). One sphincter is involuntary and the other one can stop urine flow or relax to allow it.

Rectum: The rectum lies behind the uterus and is the final part of the large intestine, which acts as a holding chamber for stool before it exits the anus. The rectum has special sensory systems to allow your body to be aware of when it needs to empty and can discern whether you have to pass gas or have a bowel movement, and how urgently.

Anus: The anus is the exit of the rectum, and also has sphincters to allow your body to void. This area is where hemorrhoids are found if you have them during pregnancy. Hemorrhoids can be internal or external.

Clitoris: The clitoris is an organ that facilitates sexual appreciation, orgasm, and is packed with nerve endings, both internally and externally. Due to the increased blood flow in the pelvis during pregnancy, many individuals experience a heightened arousal response. More on that later!

All of these organs are supported by the pelvic bones and pelvic floor muscles.

Pelvic Bones

The hip bone attaches to the...

The pelvis is composed of the ilium, ischium, and pubic bones on both sides, which are fused together and meet in the middle at the pubic symphysis in the front. You can feel the pubic symphysis with your hands: above the clitoris, under the mons pubis, or where pubic hair would lie under your underwear line.

In the back, they meet the sacral bone, which together with your coccyx (also referred to as the tailbone), form the base of your spine. This point of meeting at the pelvic bones and sacrum is the sacroiliac joint, which you can feel by those "bony dimples" in your lower back.

These bones are where the pelvic floor muscles attach. The attachment of these muscles to the pelvic bones regularly helps provide stability and have to work extra hard at this during pregnancy. However, as hormones, posture, and weight change during pregnancy, these joints can gain mobility—aka increase in motion or decrease in stability—and cause some typical, but treatable, pregnancy pains such as low back pain, sciatica, pubic symphysis dysfunction (SPD), and SI joint pain.

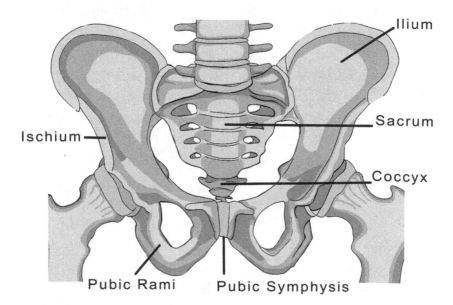

Pelvic Floor Muscles

The pelvic floor is the hammock, or lower sling of muscles, that attach to your pelvis. The pelvic floor is often referred to as the pelvic diaphragm because it is not actually a floor, but rather a functional, moving set of muscles that changes position with pressure, movements, and even your breath. These are the muscles that you feel squeeze tight when you stop your flow of urine, pinch your anus, or involuntarily contract during an orgasm.

Here's why they're useful. They:

- Provide support to the pelvic organs
- Control your bowel and bladder
- Enhance sexual function and pleasure
- Support your posture
- Stabilize your pelvis

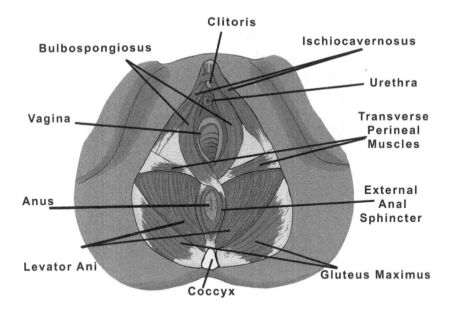

Clitoris
Bulbospongiosus
Ischiocavernosus
Urethra
Vagina
Transverse Perineal Muscles
Anus
External Anal Sphincter
Levator Ani
Gluteus Maximus
Coccyx

Quiz! Could you have pelvic floor weakness?

❑ Do you leak urine when you exercise, sneeze, cough, laugh, jump or run?

❑ Do you ever feel low-sitting pressure or heaviness in the vagina? (This may feel similar to the feeling of a tampon falling out.)

❑ Do you sometimes need to rush to the bathroom because you feel like you can't make it in time?

❑ Do you have a notion that your orgasm or climax just isn't what it could or should be?

❑ Do you feel like you go to the bathroom more than once every 90–120 minutes (excluding pregnancy)? Or plan your day around where the bathrooms might be located just in case?

If you checked "Yes" to any of the above questions, you may have some pelvic floor weakness or dysfunction that should be assessed by a pelvic floor physical therapist.

It's never wise to self-diagnose—leave it to the trained professionals when it comes to the pelvis, who can screen for other contributing issues or health concerns. In the meantime, the exercises and stretches in chapters 5 and 6 can help.

But here's an important note: although the issues above could happen because of pelvic floor weakness, they could *also* happen if your pelvic floor is too tight and not functioning correctly. Like any other muscle in the body, the pelvic floor muscles need a particular length relative to their size. Here's an easy way to understand what I mean: clench your fist into a tight ball. If your hand is stuck in that shortened, tight position, it can't open and close like it needs to grasp a coffee cup. The same applies to pelvic floor muscles: when they're too tight, they can't lengthen and shorten to create the motions needed to contract, squeeze, develop tension, or strength.

Seek out a pelvic floor physical therapist to determine what's causing problems in your case, who can address not only a weak pelvic floor, but why it is happening.

Muscles of the Inner Corset or Deep Core Muscles: The Pelvic Floor's BFFs

These muscles make up your inner corset, which help you stay upright, strong, engaged, and able to express that fierce self and belly of yours. They include:

- Your spine-stabilizing muscles
- The diaphragm
- Your lower abdominals and transverse abdominus
- The pelvic floor muscles

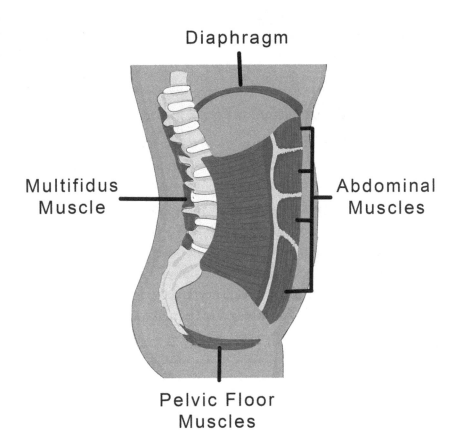

Diaphragm

Multifidus
Muscle

Abdominal
Muscles

Pelvic Floor
Muscles

As the core has become widely popularized in health and fitness, many programs neglect to educate and train the deep core muscles, including the pelvic floor. The integral system of the spinal muscles, the deep abdominals (not those six-pack muscles, sorry friends!), the pelvic floor, and your diaphragm, which allows for breath, create a dynamic system of the core. They all need each other to work and function correctly.

Here's the kicker: The deep core muscles aren't activated by traditional crunches. The good news is there are specific exercises that can help strengthen each of these key muscle groups to better support your pregnancy (jump ahead to chapter TK or keep reading!)

Quiz! Do you have a weak inner corset?

❏ Do you have chronic (long-term) mild or lower back pain?

❏ Do you ever feel unstable in your pelvis and/or lower back?

❏ Do you have difficulty getting out of bed?

❏ Do you carry your baby low during pregnancy?

❏ Do you have a tendency to waddle when you walk?

❏ Does your abdomen seem to dome out or bulge up around your belly button or the centerline of your abdomen?

❏ Do you have trouble making it to the bathroom on time? (For example, when you're running from your car to the loo—are you leaking on the way?

If you checked "yes" to any of the above, you may be dealing with some weakness in your inner corset.

Here's your next step: Hold off from buying a belly band just yet. A band can support you during pregnancy but won't provide you the strength and stability you need for laboring, pushing, delivery, or recovery. Although you may need additional support, let's work on strengthening those muscles first.

If you are doing crunches or other big ab or lifting exercises that cause your belly to dome up, take a break from that and instead work on some deep muscle strengthening before continuing those exercises. In the coming pages, I'll share key movements to try.

CHAPTER 2

Your Pelvis During Pregnancy

Hello, hormones

There are several hormones responsible for maintaining pregnancy, but one in particular can be tough to reckon with: **relaxin**. When it hits its peak at 12-14 weeks, your ligaments may become suddenly stretchy, possibly causing problems with alignment, back pain, or symphysis pubis dysfunction (AKA SPD—more on that below).

FACT CHECK: Smooth muscle is the kind of muscle that lines your organs and other areas that are involuntary—aka not under your control. That means they work without you having to think about it, and you can't stop them. Skeletal muscle is what moves us: think, quads and biceps. These your brain tells to work: to lift a coffee cup or set it down.

Hormone highlight

Here's a brief overview of the other hormone heavy hitters you've got coursing through your veins right about now.

- **Estrogen**: Estrogen is like the quarterback of pregnancy. Its role is in fetal development and uterine and breast growth.
- **Prolactin**: Prolactin assists estrogen in the development of breast tissue during pregnancy, as well as milk production. Production of this hormone is what contributes to ovulation suppression, which is why some people don't menstruate until they wean their infant from breastfeeding.
- **HCG**: Human chorionic gonadotropin is the chemical that is produced by what becomes the placenta. It tells your body that a fertilized egg is growing, alerting it to change and grow accordingly.
- **Progesterone**: This hormone's job is to relax smooth muscles (the type of muscle that surrounds your intestine and helps things to move along), particularly around the uterus. It can also contribute to relaxation of other smooth muscles. If you're newly experiencing reflux, vasodilation (lower than normal blood pressure and dizziness with standing for long periods), and constipation, progesterone is the one to thank!
- **Oxytocin**: Known as the "feel good hormone," oxytocin plays an important role in pregnancy: it helps stretch your cervix for delivery and stimulate nipples to let down milk, as well as facilitate uterine contractions. Oxytocin also contributes to bonding behaviors after birth.

⬤ Relaxin can be too...relaxing

Relaxin makes all your ligaments and tendons a little more elastic. It affects the collagen in those tissues, allowing the joints in the pelvis to separate more for birth. But this also can cause instability in joints, increasing your susceptibility to other minor injuries as well. So, plan ahead! Maximize your body's support by wearing ankle-supportive hikers if on the trail and engage your core by activating your transverse abdominus muscle (more on that below) during Zumba.

Common (but treatable!) problems during pregnancy:

You can thank the influx of relaxin, combined with changes in body shape and weight gain, for these potential issues that may pop up...

- **Sciatica:** Sometimes the sacrum can move out of place with a less stable pelvis, or a tight piriformis or other muscle that is responsible for rotating your hip can pinch your sciatic nerve. This could feel like nerve pain or a pinch sensation, burning, tingling, or numbness in that side of your butt, and may often radiate down your leg.
- **Symphysis pubis dysfunction (SPD):** Your two pubic bones come together and meet at a piece of cartilage called the pubic symphysis (under the area where you typically have pubic hair at the mons pubis). This area can become lax and misaligned causing a sharp, shooting pain that feels like it is worse when separating your legs, or standing on one leg. When excessive, SPD is most noticeable in movements like rolling in bed, side-stepping movements

like getting into the car or on a bicycle or standing on one leg like going up stairs or putting on pants.

- **Pelvic girdle pain:** The pelvic girdle consists of the ring of bones at your pelvis and the joint at which they meet. It also encompasses SPD (above). As the bones become less stable with the onset of pregnancy hormones, you may experience aching or pain with certain movements.

If you're concerned you may be showing signs of one of these issues, consult your doctor for a referral or connect with a pelvic physical therapist for a tailored treatment plan that's right for you. These are very treatable dysfunctions, and all people should have pain-free pregnancies!

*Note that this information is not intended as medical advice. Be sure to make an appointment with your OB/GYN to discuss any pelvic pain you're experiencing.

 Too weak...or too tight?

Pelvic floor dysfunction can be a result of weakness—but weakness doesn't always mean that your body can't contract well. It could also mean that your muscles are too strong or tight, so they can't relax fully to develop a substantive contraction. Fear not! Weak muscles can be trained to be stronger, and tight muscles can be trained to elongate to hold strong against pressure (i.e., not leak when you jump), as well as relax fully (i.e., to birth vaginally or have a bowel movement).

Diving into Diastasis Recti

One of the top questions I get asked by someone who is expecting is how to prevent abdominal separation—or diastasis recti (DR). During pregnancy, diastasis recti is a normal separation of the muscular abdominal wall (rectus abdominus muscles) along the midline (linea alba), running from below your sternum to above your pubic bones.

Not familiar with the linea alba? Pretend you're drawing a line from just below your breastbone, down through your belly button, and down to your lower pubic line, or where your pubic hair would begin. That is the linea alba, or that thick tendon sheath where the muscles of your right side meet your left. DR might sound scary, but in reality, your muscles themselves aren't actually coming apart from themselves. Instead, they are pulling and separating away from the long tendon where they meet along the centerline of your abdomen. Diastasis recti can occur along part of the midline or all of it, and varies in depth and width by individual. Ideally, we can minimize this during pregnancy and avoid actions that worsen it.

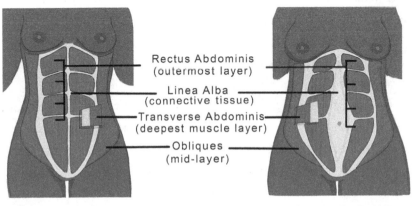

Rectus Abdominis
(outermost layer)

Linea Alba
(connective tissue)

Transverse Abdominis
(deepest muscle layer)

Obliques
(mid-layer)

Normal Abdomen   Diastasis Recti

Should you worry about it?

Diastasis recti is **normal** to make space for the growing baby in your belly! How much your muscles separate from the midline is related to various physiological reasons, such as our good friend relaxin, plus your underlying strength, size, genetics, previous medical history, and other factors that are mostly out of your control. Genetics in particular determine how your collagen responds to stretching and contractions, as collagen is the main component of stretch tissue in ligaments and tendons. This is also why some people get stretch marks and others do not.

Here's the kicker: this separation may not close up or return to normal postpartum and varies by person. My advice: watch, prevent, and **don't** excessively worry.

You may start to see that when you flex your abdominals, roll in bed, sit up, or lift heavy things, the tissue along the center of your abdomen domes up. Alternatively, you might feel a gap with your fingers starting around your navel.

However fairly normal, there can be too much of a good thing. If the space is getting *too* wide, it may be an indication that you need to modify your activity. Common causes for abdominal doming include regularly lifting heavy things (like an older toddler) or exercise such as crunches. Additionally, if you feel like you're carrying your pregnancy really low, these are potential signs of weakness and poor abdominal muscle control.

Ideally, you want to be evaluated and educated on how to best contract your deep inner corset muscles so that you can prevent exacerbation of diastasis recti. This will help strengthen your inner support system and allow you to do the exercises you love (safely). These things will help prevent low back pain, prevent SPD and pelvic girdle pain, and facilitate an easier and speedier recovery postpartum.

What to do if you think you might have DR

Resist the urge to self-diagnose or go down the internet rabbit hole. It's not uncommon for me to see people in my clinical practice that have avoided any exercise due to fear of DR—but this is the opposite of what I want! Movement and exercise help regulate mood, blood pressure, swelling, weight, and blood sugar. It helps with optimal positioning of the baby, improves muscle tone, and prepares you for birth, amongst other benefits.

First, put a hold on exercises or movements that cause your belly to dome or bulge up along the centerline. This might mean taking to your knees during some yoga poses, getting out of bed by rolling to the side, or asking for a hand when unloading groceries. Next, contact a pelvic physical therapist to get specific exercises, movement techniques, and other supportive tips to assist your abdominal muscles and core pressure during pregnancy to help reduce further separation and optimize the closure of the DR postpartum.

Pelvic physical therapy for DR during pregnancy

A pelvic physical therapist will do a full evaluation first. They will ask about your exercise history, what you enjoy doing for movement, your work life/activity, and address any bowel/bladder/pelvic concerns. They will also do a detailed examination of your core, pelvic floor, and hip muscle strength, function, and skeletal alignment during pregnancy. It is important to share your goals and work together to establish a plan of care that reflects your needs and goals based on your input and their findings and recommendations. Goals might include things like continuing to run through your pregnancy, lift weights, work as a flight attendant and lift luggage regularly, etc.

In the case of abdominal weakness or diastasis recti, your pelvic physical therapist may prescribe muscle-strengthening exercises or releases or work on correcting the alignment of your pelvis. They may choose to utilize methods of taping or other support garments or suggest postural and movement changes specific to your needs. Every body is different! In many cases, a little pelvic education on how to move and breathe differently can change how you exercise and mindfully support your abdominal control so you can keep doing what you love throughout pregnancy comfortably.

DR is super common!

Diastasis recti usually happens in the later stages of pregnancy and may get worse in your second or subsequent pregnancies. However, people who have never been pregnant can have DR too! That's why it's so crucial to strengthen those deep abdominal muscles of your inner corset.

Research says: DR frequency

"DRA occurs most frequently during pregnancy and regresses spontaneously after childbirth in most women. However, at 12 months postpartum, 33% of women still experience DRA [6]. DRA has been found in 39% of older, parous women undergoing abdominal hysterectomy [7], and in 52% of urogynecological menopausal patients [8], suggesting that DRA can even persist past childbearing years. Data from nonparturient women are rare. Diastasis is also frequently present in men, but data regarding these cases are scarce." (Cavalli et al., 2021)

PART 2:

PREPARING YOUR PELVIS

CHAPTER 3:

Pelvic Floor Contractions

Work that pelvic floor

To kegel or not to kegel?

Pelvic floor muscle contractions, commonly referred to as kegels, are often over-prescribed and are not right for everyone. Put simply, pelvic floor contractions are used to strengthen your pelvic floor muscles. Indications that these muscles may be weak, or not doing their job as they should, include leaking urine or feces, pelvic organ prolapse, weak orgasms, and poor core strength.

However, sometimes leaking or having a poor ability to contract these muscles is actually a sign that they are TOO tight and can't relax, as mentioned earlier. Muscles can be both tight and weak or too lengthened and weak—so read on before you do all those pelvic squeezes!

If you have a history of pain during sex or insertion of a tampon, tailbone pain, or other pelvic pain, I highly encourage you to connect with a pelvic physical therapist to see if pelvic floor contractions are right for you. In some cases, it may benefit you more to work on relaxation and breathing techniques instead.

Benefits of learning how to contract (and relax) these muscles:

- Improved coordination and awareness, which will be helpful during active birth and pushing when you are trying to relax and open these muscle groups
- Improved strength and endurance of the muscles
- Increased blood flow to the pelvis
- Improved sexual function (orgasm, blood flow and control)
- Improved athletic outcomes (we're talking to you, runners and CrossFitters!)

You should talk to a provider if you check *any* of these boxes...

❏ Sex, penetration, or insertion of a menstrual cup or tampon is painful.

❏ You feel heaviness or bulging, similar to a sensation that a tampon is falling out or see bulging of tissue at the opening of your vagina when you look with a hand mirror.

❏ You leak stool, or you feel like after you wipe, there's more still coming out—or you feel unclean or see underwear staining later even after wiping well.

❏ You have a traumatic past sexual experience or event and doing pelvic floor exercises is triggering.

How to do a pelvic floor contraction:

First, let's find your pelvic floor.

Try either laying down with your legs supported and relaxed or sitting upright. We want your pelvic floor to do the work—not your glutes or leg muscles.

Inhale deeply, letting your belly fill with air and expand. Feel the pelvic floor gently expand and lengthen. Think of it like a tight budded flower that is now blossoming. As you then gently exhale, contract, like you're holding back urine or gas.

You should feel both your outer vulvar and anorectal area gently pinch and lift up and in. This is your pelvic floor!

Repeat this movement with deep breathing five times.

Start slowly

Begin doing pelvic floor contractions laying down (it's the easiest position to engage your pelvic floor) and progress to sitting, standing, and during regular exercise and movement. Your pelvic floor has to operate all the time (it's so busy!) to react to your movements and changes, like a jump or a sneeze.

When you're just starting out, focus on just **five contractions plus breathing, 4-5 times per day.** Once that becomes second nature, progress to **two sets of ten, twice per day**—but don't overdo it. Doing hundreds of pelvic floor contractions, especially if you aren't doing them correctly, won't do you any additional good. Instead, it may cause more discomfort or over-tightening of these muscles. During your third trimester especially, pelvic floor *relaxation* is just as important as pelvic floor strength.

Your partner can join in too! All bodies have a pelvic floor. If your partner has a penis, it feels like raising the penis and testicles.

Remember: never hold your breath or bear down with your abs as if you were straining to have a bowel movement. Don't be the Hulk! This should be gentle. Some weightlifters brace their abdomen and hold their breath during lifting. Don't do that, especially during pregnancy. Bearing down while holding your breath can force downward pressure onto your pelvic organs, like your bladder and uterus, which can cause pelvic organ prolapse, pelvic floor dysfunction, etc.

Progress

Once you feel like you've got the contraction mastered while laying down, then sitting, try doing it standing. An easy way to start is by standing and putting your hands flat on a countertop, while leaning slightly forward. Feel your pelvic floor engage—you might also feel some subtle core engagement. Try to dissuade your glutes and thigh muscles from kicking in—can you isolate the feeling? Be mindful of not holding your breath or "gripping" your muscles in your abdomen or thighs while in this position.

The history of the kegel

Pelvic floor health has been referenced and alluded to since ancient times. Awareness of this muscle group is nothing new but was seemingly forgotten by modern medicine until the term kegel was coined by Dr. Arnold Kegel, who published research in 1948 on the pelvic floor contraction in the 1940s. However, one of the true founders of modern pelvic health was Margaret Morris.

Morris was a former dancer turned physical therapist who practiced, researched, and published work in the 1930s on the integration of breath, movement, and posture during labor and delivery. Her work in the UK, published as "Maternity and Post Operative Exercises in Diagrams and Words" was released in 1937. However, thanks to common cultural gender biases of that era, Morris' work gained substantially less recognition.

As Dr. Kegel launched forward with his own research and publications on pelvic floor strengthening exercises to facilitate continence in women, his name became synonymous with the kegel. His research and exercises were more detailed than today's simplified version of the self-taught kegel, but essentially helped draw awareness to methods of strengthening the pelvic floor muscles to assist patients with pelvic organ prolapse and incontinence—dysfunctions that previously were largely left untreated or ignored.

CHAPTER 4:

Exercise & Movement

Whether, when, and how

All About Exercise

E xercise during pregnancy is very personal and can be emotionally charged. For many people, the kind of exercise they do—whether a weekly yoga routine, distance running, or a membership to a Crossfit cube—is a part of their identity. It can also provide a sense of belonging to a community.

Making any blanket statement about exercise during pregnancy would be flawed: for those that have had any prior complications or are high-risk, it is always advised to seek clearance from your medical provider for the kinds of exercise you wish to perform. But for the general population, the American Academy of Obstetricians and Gynecologists (ACOG) advises people that they may continue performing any exercise they are already doing, but to avoid starting a new kind of exercise.

Layman's terms? If you weren't a runner before, now is not the time to start. Enjoy easy three-mile runs in the morning and are still feeling good? Keep at it. Use your body and how you feel as a barometer, and never hesitate to reach out to your medical care team, midwife, or pelvic physical therapist for advice or recommendations.

Once your care provider clears you for exercise, it's definitely time to get moving. Exercising during pregnancy leads to loads of benefits for your body and baby (more below). Experts recommend a minimum of 2.5 hours of moderate-intensity aerobic exercise each week—low-impact activities like walking and swimming are ideal.

 What is moderate-intensity exercise?

Moderate-intensity exercise is defined as aerobic exercise (aka, gets your heart rate up) that gets you moving and sweating, enough so that you can talk but not necessarily sing the words to your favorite song.

Beyond getting your heart pumping and blood flowing, it's also important to develop a specific set of muscles during pregnancy. Building (or maintaining) strength in these targeted muscle groups is essential, because when there's weakness in your inner core or pelvic floor muscles, it could result in pain or continence issues (read: leakage) now or down the line.

Physical activity is also essential to developing the strength and endurance that will allow you to safely and effectively hold different positions—like a deep squat—during labor. You wouldn't compete in a triathlon without training first, right? That's exactly what we're going to start doing right now. These exercises are gentle enough that even if you are an activity newbie, they're safe to perform.

8 great reasons to exercise throughout pregnancy

Regular physical activity...

1. Improves blood flow and vascularity (it brings the good stuff in and sends the bad stuff out), while keeping your heart, lungs and blood vessels in good working order.

2. Improves posture, helping to stave off low back pain or neck strain as your body's center of gravity shifts forward with a growing belly. It also helps with the position of the baby towards the end of pregnancy.

3. Boosts the support system for abdominal and pelvic organs, easing some of the discomfort during pregnancy.

4. Helps prevent some birth-related injuries and traumas and reduces the risk of complications like preeclampsia (high blood pressure during pregnancy) or gestational diabetes.

5. Releases happy, feel-good hormones like dopamine and serotonin (the brain's mood boosters), as well as endorphins, which provide a natural "kick" to your system that also acts as an analgesic (pain reliever). Who doesn't want an additional happy boost during pregnancy?

6. Allows opening through the pelvic floor muscles and relaxation through the hips, facilitating optimal positioning, descent, and vaginal delivery of your baby. Exercise during pregnancy may reduce the need for a Cesarean section.

7. Increases your comfort and confidence, meaning you'll experience less pain during pregnancy and feel more in control of your body and movements as you approach labor and delivery.

8. It benefits baby too! As you move, your body uses stores of fat and glucose more efficiently, helping baby stay a healthy size. Your mood also affects your baby, and there

is mounting evidence indicating that movement during pregnancy may increase your baby's interest and motivation to move and exercise once they are earthside.

Need more examples?

Exercise also facilitates easy and healthy bowel movements, helps reduce swelling that's common in pregnancy, and is a fun activity you can do to relieve anxiety or stress alone or with a friend or partner.

Exercising with morning sickness

Been there, done that, and it is certainly not fun. Truth be told, my running partner was the first friend of mine to find out I was pregnant when I rounded a corner and stuck my head into a bush to vomit during a run, very early on in my pregnancy. The surging hormones of the first trimester can be a rough ride for many people, so never force yourself to exercise and mentally cut yourself some slack if you can't stick to your normal routine.

Your body is undergoing the greatest physiological change it possibly can, and that takes a lot of work. Scheduling naps and rest breaks may be as critical as scheduling exercise during these months. If you do have morning sickness, exercise can benefit by releasing hormones that aid your body's response to stressors and fatigue, but also help your body to process all those extra pregnancy hormones floating around.

Always consult your doctor or medical care team if you are experiencing severe morning sickness, dehydration, weight loss, dizziness, or other symptoms prior to exercise during pregnancy.

Tips for exercising with morning sickness:

1. Track when you feel your best throughout the day, versus when you feel most nauseated or fatigued, and change your workout time to match your "best."

2. Eat small bites of food throughout the day between regular meals as well as staying well hydrated.

3. Never force it: some days require naps or a change in type of exercise.

4. Ask your midwife or doula! These integral members of the birth support community have tons of resources for staving off the nausea related to the rise in hormones, from wrist bands to ginger or mint. Having some power players in your kitchen or bathroom to tag team your other efforts are helpful.

5. Deep diaphragmatic breathing (belly breathing) or meditation with yogi breath helps your brain to reroute off the nausea, with the added benefit of relaxation.

6. Change your workout clothes. Loose, baggy clothes around the midsection may feel better during these early days.

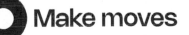 **Make moves**

I get it. We aren't all taking a daily 6am spin session or leaning into a 5-mile run after work. Movement, as I define it, is creating motion at your joints, using your muscles to drive you into that motion, elevating your heart rate, and grounding your spirit. Movement on a daily basis doesn't have to mean you have to invest in fancy exercise equipment. It can mean taking a walk with your best bipedal or four-legged friend, getting up from your office chair for a 5-minute stretch break between calls, cleaning your kitchen, gardening, or mowing your lawn. Creating routines that make your body and mind feel good now will help with the sometimes-isolating period of the fourth trimester (or initial three-month postpartum period) and will also encourage your little one to move their body as they see you doing it. Ditch the idea of a traditional "workout" if it doesn't speak to you—and get creative with how you can make moves in your daily routine.

The Pelvic Prep School Circuit

There are many different kinds of exercise, but when it comes to exercise during pregnancy, there are three simple parts: aerobic, strengthening, and stretching. As a busy, working mom-to-be, I needed a concise, easy to follow plan to maximize my time and reward that incorporated all three of these parts. The exercises in the circuit below, combined with individually preferred aerobic activity, have had the most impact for the vast majority of my clients (and me!).

These should primarily be started in the second trimester and continued into the third, while the stretches can be used through-out all three trimesters. Find the photos and how-to's starting on page TK. All together, the exercises should take about 15 minutes, and the stretches should take about 10 minutes.

One thing most people tend to forget while pregnant is that you're growing a new person—but this is a time to take care of yourself too! The time spent on yourself now will repay you in dividends by supporting a better sense of calm, control, and ability to focus. This will also create a structured, healthy routine that can carry you through postpartum, recovery, return to work, exercise, and other parts of pre-baby life you're eager to return to.

THE PELVIC PREP SCHOOL CIRCUIT

EXERCISE	REP	FREQUENCY
Abdominal Engagement	Two sets of 10–12	Daily to every other day
Clamshells	Two sets of 10–12	Daily to every other day
Bird Dogs	Two sets of 15–20	Daily to every other day
Bridges	Two sets of 10–12	Daily to every other day
Wall Squats	Two sets of 10–12	Daily to every other day

STRETCH	REP	FREQUENCY
Deep Squat	Hold for 30 seconds, repeat three times	Once daily
Happy Baby	Hold for 30 seconds, repeat three times	Once daily
Supported Butterfly	Hold for 30 seconds, repeat three times	Once daily
The Figure-4	Hold for 30 seconds, repeat three times	Once daily
Cat-Cow	Hold for 30 seconds, repeat three times	Once daily
Child's Pose	Hold for 30 seconds, repeat three times	Once daily

⬤ Don't skip the basics

I regularly treat elite athletes—including Olympic medal-winning runners and CrossFit champions—who demonstrate significant speed, endurance, and strength. But when I test their deep abdominal muscles, hip muscles, or pelvic floor, I often find significant weakness. Surprised? Here's why: many exercise programs or traditional training techniques emphasize our big, global "mover muscles," which help in strength and speed and build muscle bulk. But working the deeper muscle layers, which stabilize and control movement, is often left out of training—possibly because these muscles are much more difficult to cue and identify weakness without understanding the systems. So, remember: even if you are performing high-level fitness, take a step back and make sure to learn to engage these basics.

First Trimester

For most individuals, the first trimester is likely a continuation of exercise or movement you've already been doing, whether that's running, walking, yoga, spinning, swimming, weightlifting, CrossFit, or something else. The name of the game is to maintain.

A reminder that ACOG recommends pregnant persons remain active throughout pregnancy and continue to exercise (barring physical conditions or specific advice to the contrary from a medical provider) with the same routines they were doing prior to becoming pregnant.

In a nutshell, if your pre-pregnancy exercise routines are still working for you, keep going! Just listen to your body and back off on the intensity or duration if need be. If you're not able to keep up with your previous routines (thanks, hormones), or if you haven't yet found a form of movement you love, consider adding low-impact exercise like walking, yoga or swimming. Check out our faves on page TK.

If you are considered to have a high-risk pregnancy, have extreme morning sickness, placenta previa, preeclampsia, or another physical condition, movement during pregnancy may look very different for you—don't be shy about getting personalized advice from your healthcare team.

The information and exercises contained in this book are not a substitute for medical advice. You should seek counsel from your pelvic physical therapist, OB/GYN, or midwife prior to beginning any exercise routine. ACOG recommends not starting a new exercise while pregnant: so, if you weren't a runner or heavy lifter before, now is **<u>NOT</u>** the time to start.

FIRST TRIMESTER: DAY-AT-A-GLANCE

The Goal: In the first few months, aim to move and stretch your body in whatever way feels good to you. As you progress, the focus shifts to aligning the body for birth, training your breath, and preparing your body for the "aftershocks" of birth—recovering postpartum. And remember, your exercise timing will also depend on whether you are experiencing morning sickness or fatigue: Trust your gut and give your body rest and nourishment when it seeks it.

Good to Know: Avoid exercising on an empty stomach: Your body needs fuel to move, so a light snack 20 to 30 minutes before your morning exercise is smart. You may continue your current strength training program, however, listen to your body. If something doesn't feel right, it's probably not right for you right now.

MORNING:

- Start with a five-minute mindful meditation: manifest what the day looks like for you, envision your baby growing, and connect with your pregnancy body. I recommend doing these while laying on your left side, with a pillow between your knees, or in a supported sitting position. Choose a guided meditation or listen to calming music, practicing deep, diaphragmatic breathwork. *Try this daily.*

- Follow with 10-30 min of moderate-intensity cardio exercise, like speed walking, jogging, swimming, or cycling on a stationary bike. Make sure to spend five minutes cooling down afterward (a slow walk is ideal.) Your body is adjusting to an increase in blood volume, which means your heart is working hard to pump that extra fluid—give it time to recover. *Try this 4-5 days a week or what feels comfortable to you.*

MIDDAY:

- Take a few five-minute stretch breaks between morning and midday, especially if you spend a lot of your day seated. *Try this daily.*

LUNCH:

- Go for a 10-15 min walk with your co-workers, kids, or to just pop out for some sunshine. *Try this 3-5 times per week.*

AFTERNOON:

- Take a few five-minute stretch breaks between midday and the early evening, especially if you spend a lot of your day seated. *Try this daily.*

EVENING:

- Use our full stretch circuit to wind down, followed by five minutes of breath work. If you practice yoga nidra or prenatal yoga, this is a great time to incorporate those practices. *Try this daily.*

Don't Sweat It

If you can't commit to doing all of this daily, don't stress. Even following this plan just two or three times a week will result in major benefits. You'll begin to tune in with your body more and learn what feels right (or wrong), tight, strong or weak. Some days you might only squeeze in a morning meditation and a stretch break or two, and that's OK! Or maybe you can only fit in a workout on the weekends. Figure out whatever works for you.

Second Trimester

Often the favorite trimester, when fatigue subsides, and morning sickness abates. For the lucky ones, you've got that pregnancy hormone glow and might start to pop your bump! You're also likely experiencing more of an energy boost during these months, and now's a great time to start really strengthening the specific muscle sets that'll help you prepare for labor and birth. Try to incorporate the Pelvic Prep School Circuit daily or at least a few times per week, and when these moves get too easy, reach out to a pelvic physical therapist for a progression of more targeted exercises and continued care into your third trimester.

As your belly starts to get a little bigger, some exercise routines may begin to feel a bit uncomfortable or require more modifications. If you're practicing yoga, for example, make sure to find a prenatal-friendly class or ask your teacher for specific poses you should modify or avoid when pregnant.

We recommend keeping up with 30 minutes per day of light- to moderate-intensity movement, if and when you can, and as long as you're still feeling good. This is also a great time to continue your current lifting program, remembering to keep your transverse abdominis and lower abdominals engaged. Combined with good body mechanics and breathwork, these will also help prevent diastasis recti and lower back pain.

SECOND TRIMESTER: DAY–AT–A–GLANCE

The Goal: By now your morning sickness is creeping off, your energy is rebounding, and you may or may not be sporting a baby bump. The second trimester is a great time to move and really start to strengthen those muscles that'll help train your body for labor and help with delivery. You can incorporate the circuit exercises listed in the chart above now, too.

Good to Know: You'll still want to eat a light meal (a smoothie or a protein bar rich in seed or nut butters are good options) before working out, but don't go for anything too heavy—your digestive organs are starting to be pushed up a little higher...which can sometimes mean reflux. And thanks to relaxin, your lower esophageal sphincter may be relaxed, too, also contributing to reflux during this stage.

MORNING:

- Start with a five-minute mindful meditation: manifest what the day looks like for you, envision your baby growing, and connect with your pregnancy body. I recommend doing these while laying on your left side, with a pillow between your knees, or in a supported sitting position. Choose a guided meditation or listen to calming music, practicing deep, diaphragmatic breathwork we've instructed you in. *Try this daily.*

- Follow with 10-30 minutes of moderate-intensity cardio exercise, like speed walking, jogging, swimming, or cycling on a stationary bike. Moderate intensity means you're getting your heart rate up but can still have a conversation. Cool down, then go into our exercise circuit of 5 exercises. *Try this 4-5 days a week or what feels comfortable to you.*

MIDDAY:

- Take a few five-minute stretch breaks between morning and midday, especially if you spend a lot of your day seated. *Try this daily.*

LUNCH:

- Go for a 10-15 min walk with your co-workers, kids or to just pop out for some sunshine. *Try this 3-5 times per week.*

AFTERNOON:

- Take a few five-minute stretch breaks between midday and the early evening, especially if you spend a lot of your day seated. *Try this daily.*

EVENING:

- Use our full exercise and stretch circuit to wind down, followed by five minutes of breath work. If you practice yoga nidra or prenatal yoga, this is a great time to incorporate those practices. *Try this daily.*

Third Trimester

The final countdown has begun: you've entered the third trimester, you're feeling more at ease in pregnancy, and you're preparing for labor and birth. By now, your bump is leading you into rooms, your movement may have slowed, and even getting out of bed might feel different (or harder!)

The third trimester should focus on a combination of strengthening, stretching, and relaxation to prepare for delivery. The primary goal is to elongate the pelvic floor—or help it relax—while also keeping up with strength. Keep up with your stretches, and try to incorporate more deep breathing work too, which will pay off greatly during labor and birth. Now is also a great time to connect with a pelvic physical therapist for additional customized strengthening exercises and variations to your current aerobic exercise, as states of ability can vary greatly during this stage.

Maintain your regular physical activity during this time as best you can, making sure that your expanding belly stays supported. You may need to employ the use of things like belly bands and compression socks during this stage. If you feel any pressure or pain, stop what you're doing and immediately inform your care provider.

THIRD TRIMESTER: DAY–AT–A–GLANCE

The Goal: Keep it up but take things slowly and back off as needed. You may be slowing down a little in general. As your uterus expands and your baby grows, you may feel shortness of breath, as there's suddenly less room for your diaphragm to drop and your lungs to expand to fill with air. Make sure to take breaks when you need to and listen to your body.

Good to Know: Third trimester is a great time to see a pelvic physical therapist, especially if you participate in high impact sports such as running or do heavy lifting. Both of these activities create downward pressure on your pelvic floor, so you'll want to ensure that your pelvic floor is a) strong enough to counter that impact; and b) not tightening too much as a result of fending off that impact. Now is the time we want you to start opening, relaxing, and preparing your pelvic floor for delivery.

MORNING:

- Start with a five-minute mindful meditation: manifest what the day looks like for you, envision your baby growing, and connect with your pregnancy body. I recommend doing these while laying on your left side, with a pillow between your knees, or in a supported sitting position. Choose a guided meditation or listen to calming music, practicing deep, diaphragmatic breathwork. *Try this daily.*
- Follow with cat/cow stretches to get your blood flowing and your body moving pre-exercise. Then, do 15-20 minutes of moderate-intensity cardio exercise, like brisk walking, or moderate resistance indoor cycling. Moderate intensity means you're getting your heart rate up but can still have a conversation. Cool down, then go into the Pelvic School Prep Course exercise circuit. *Try this 4-5 days a week or what feels comfortable to you.*

MIDDAY:

- Take a few five-minute stretch breaks between morning and midday, especially if you spend a lot of your day seated. *Try this daily.*

LUNCH:

- Go for a 10-15 min walk with your co-workers, kids or to just pop out for some sunshine. *Try this 3-5 times per week.*

AFTERNOON:

- Take a few five-minute stretch breaks between midday and the early evening, especially if you spend a lot of your day seated. *Try this daily.*

EVENING:

- Use our full exercise and stretch circuit to wind down, followed by 5 minutes of breath work. If you practice yoga nidra or prenatal yoga, this is a great time to incorporate those practices. *Try this daily.*

EXERCISES HOW-TO

First, a reminder: none of the exercises or stretches should be painful. You may feel the muscles activating—or firing up—but there should be no actual pain. Pain can be sudden, sharp, shooting, dull/aching, and occur while at rest and/or during exercise. If there is, see your care provider!

Exercise 1: Abdominal Engagement

Your deep abdominals, specifically the transverse abdominis muscle, start at your spine and wrap around you like a corset, going from the bottom of your sternum to your pubic bone. This muscle is responsible for stabilizing the pressure in your abdomen, balance, proper posture, and alignment, and so much more. It's also an essential muscle during lifting, which you'll be doing a lot of—roughly 35 pounds regularly with your baby and a car seat!

Fun fact: The transverse abdominis is my favorite muscle (you know, if I had to pick).

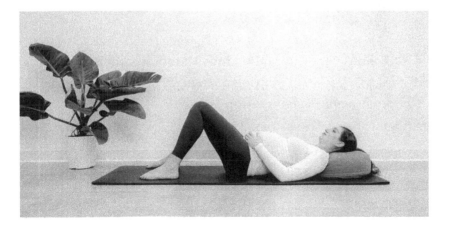

1. Start in a comfortable position—either on your back propped slightly with a pillow or seated with a lumbar support—with relaxed and bent knees to slacken the abdomen. Try to keep your low back in neutral: you don't want too much curving, so remind yourself to slightly flatten it. Bending your knees will help. During the second and third trimester, we don't want you flat on your back, as the pressure from the placenta and growing baby can restrict returning blood flow and make you woozy. Prop up!

2. Brace yourself, literally: slowly inhale, filling your belly with air. Then, on an exhale, think about gently drawing your belly button in towards your spine, or hugging the baby inward.

3. Repeat this sequence; but this time, think about drawing not only your belly in, but also gently engaging the muscles along your spine.

4. Continue to repeat. Think about keeping your ribs pointed down and your posture upright (no crunching right now).

5. Don't hold your breath. Visualize an inhale, full belly, exhale, engage, and repeat 10-12 times. Repeat this 2-3 times throughout the day.

Check in with your body: Once you master the technique in this position, try it while sitting or standing. We want this muscle to work no matter what position you are in—it's helping to hold your baby!

Exercise 2: Clamshells

This exercise strengthens your hip external rotator muscles, which assist the pelvic floor and do lots of work during labor for positioning.

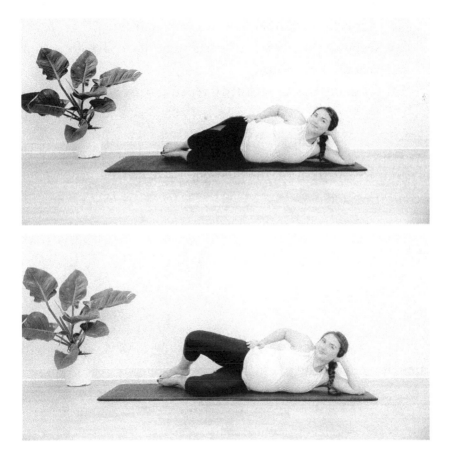

1. Start by lying down on your side. Keep ankles together and separate your knees, like a clam opening. You should feel this position working the muscles in the area where the back pocket of your jeans normally hits; if not, adjust the angle of your hips to bring your knees either closer to your belly, or further down toward your feet.
2. Keep your hips "stacked" straight up/down. Try not to roll back onto your hips.
3. Try doing this as a set of 10 repetitions.

Check in with your body: too easy? Add a few repetitions and/or a resistance band above your knees. Ideally, you should be able to perform two sets of 15-20 repetitions properly by the end of the second trimester.

Exercise 3: Bird Dogs

Strengthen your deep abdominal, pelvic, spinal, and postural muscles—and help all those friends work together in a community of pelvic love.

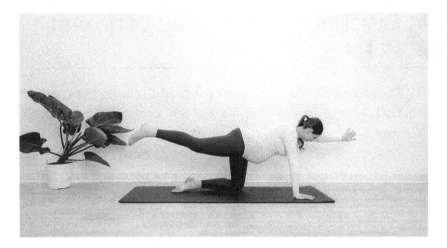

1. Begin on your hands and knees on your yoga mat. Your hands can be flat against the mat, or in fists if it is more comfortable for your wrists.
2. Take a normal breath: inhale to prep your system, then exhale and use the engagement of your transverse abdominus muscles to hold your pelvis in a neutral position while you extend one leg and the opposite arm straight out. Then, bring them in to return to all fours.
3. Alternate sides with your breath, with a focus on keeping your pelvis neutral and stable while your arms and legs move. Try for two sets of 15-20 repetitions.

Check in with your body: You should feel your core holding you steady while you move, meaning you should notice your butt muscles (glutes) firing to kick your leg back. Are you noticing a wobbly middle section? Work with your breath: inhale, exhale, engage, move. This helps all the parts of the core muscles work together to integrate a stable system while you move dynamically.

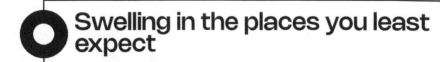

Swelling in the places you least expect

Pregnancy can be hard on your wrists. Crossing the inside of your wrist is a narrow canal full of tendons for all the muscles that flex your fingers and wrist. Normally there is just enough space around these slippery tendons to slide and glide across each other. But with fluid retention and swelling during pregnancy, this little canal can tighten up with less free space to move and glide. As a result, this can cause carpal tunnel syndrome during pregnancy. Bracing, taping, good posture during computer work, and using fisted hands in lieu of flat palms during certain exercises can help.

Exercise 4: Bridges

This exercise works your glutes—a big powerhouse in your body that also helps hold you in different positions needed for laboring. That means that having endurance in these muscles is super important.

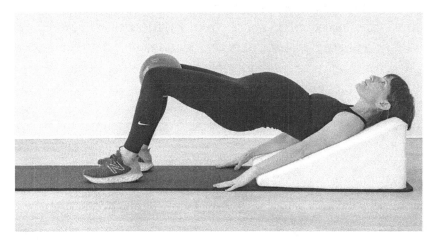

1. Start by laying on your back if you are early in pregnancy or propped up with a pillow or your yoga bolster, arms down at your side.
2. Lift your hips up and squeeze your butt, staying low enough so that you don't roll back up onto your neck. Try to keep your spine neutral instead of tucking your butt.
3. Do two sets of 10, holding for 10 seconds each repetition. Want to add difficulty? Try doing a pelvic floor contraction and holding it while you're up there.

Check in with your body: Make sure you're really engaging your butt muscles while trying to quiet your hamstrings. Want to make it even more challenging? Add a yoga block between your knees and squeeze that along with your glutes as you rise up.

"Mom butt" is real

The tilt of your pelvis during pregnancy can alter the ability of your glutes to contract and fire like they used to. Paired with hormonal changes, this can lead to that "flat butt" that my clients often complain about. Fear not, friends! Exercising your glutes both during and after pregnancy can get your booty poppin' again. It isn't all for looks: these muscles are super important for walking, getting up hills or stairs, running, and stabilizing the load your body takes on as it moves through space.

Exercise 5: Squats

Work that tush! This do-anywhere exercise gives more love to the glutes, which tend to lose their oomph during pregnancy and immediately postpartum.

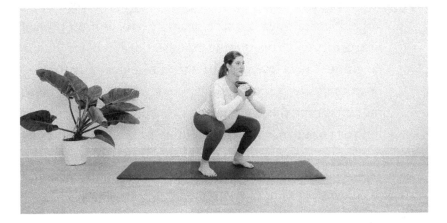

1. Stand with your feet hip-width apart, or you can lean up against an exercise ball against the wall, starting with the ball along your low back.
2. Inhale going down. As you come up, blow out through your lips and push through your heels to feel your butt activate. You can keep your arms to the side or out in front of you.
3. Remember: your knees should follow an imaginary vertical line rising from your second toe, and never go past that line. Hinge at your hips.
4. Start with two sets of 10. How does that feel? Add 5-10 repetitions to each set, or a third set. Remember, the quality is important here. You should feel your glutes and breath working!

Check in with your body: Too easy? Hold a kettlebell, weighted ball, or free weight in front of you.

More Ways to Move

In addition to the five exercises you've just learned, it's also a great idea to work in other opportunities for safe movement. Once your doctor or midwife approves you for exercise, try these... (All incorporate hip, pelvic and core strengthening...plus relaxation!)

- **Yoga**: Prenatal yoga is my pregnancy go-to, as most trained instructors will have specific modifications in place. Prenatal group classes (even virtual ones) are a great way to meet other pregnant parents and help to develop a sense of community during this big transition time. Remember to avoid hot yoga or intense stretching during pregnancy. Your body is already laxer due to that nagging friend relaxin, so no pretzels, please. I love the added bonus of mindfulness and connection to your body and baby that yoga adds.

- **Pilates**: The reformer is a helpful tool in stretching and coordinating core to lower body movements with your breath and deep abdominals. I can't say enough good things about a Pilates class with an instructor well-versed in prenatal modifications. From balance to stretching, upper body to lower, a reformer workout is very inclusive. Avoid crunch-like actions without guidance. As with any exercise, if it causes your abdomen to "dome up" it should be avoided. Seek out care for diastasis recti prevention and to learn how to engage your deep core muscles with your breath to more appropriately control the pressure in your abdomen.

- **Barre**: Barre is a great way to build strength, stretch, and move your body, all in one session.

- **Dance**: Free-form dance sessions allow for an expression of self, emotion, and physical freedom. We love letting the belly move and flow and finding a new rhythm under your feet.

A Word on Walking

Walking is my favorite pregnancy go-to. Try to incorporate it daily, in the form of 2-3 10-minute strolls. Walking helps:

- Ease morning sickness and fatigue
- Regulate blood sugar
- Stimulate blood flow to the pelvis
- Reduce ankle and lower leg swelling
- Release the positive endorphins from your brain

A Note to Runners

Yes, many of you can keep pounding that pavement—but to do it safely, there are many factors you need to consider. Running is an impact sport. The impact varies based on your form, the type of material you run on (trails versus pavement, etc.), bodyweight, biomechanics and other factors. Physics is your friend!

A growing belly means your center of mass—or how your weight is distributed and supported by your body—shifts forward. In turn, this alters your running dynamics. Running also isn't right for everyone during pregnancy. For some people, I recommend something lower impact, such as swimming, water aerobics, or a spin bike. Water jogging with a swim belt encourages maintenance of cardiovascular fitness and running-like fitness without impact, with the added benefit of the hydrostatic pressure of water. In layman's terms, this means it can help decrease swelling.

Runners, by definition, are a broad group of body types, ages, running abilities and levels, with varying health considerations. A considerable amount of research has been and continues to be compiled, in efforts to best determine strategy and outcomes for running during and after pregnancy. From footwear changes due to increased body mass and possible foot size and arch changes, to support garments like prenatal running sports bras and compression tights, to an increased hydration and nutrition needs, running during pregnancy often requires adaptations.

If you're a runner, I strongly urge you to consult with professionals across the spectrum that suit your particular needs. You may also want to consider working with a pelvic physical therapist who has experience working with pregnant runners to maximize your biomechanics and form as your body changes. Most importantly, you should work with someone who is credentialed and can provide personalized recommendations for keeping you—and your pelvic organs—safe.

Admittedly, we all toe the line here: of course, we want to promote feminism, the ability and badass strength and determination of pregnant runners and competitors, and support postpartum athletes. But there is also a right way to do it. Strength and ferocity aren't measured by how far into your pregnancy you continue running or how quickly you return. Taking the appropriate steps along the way will facilitate both of these aspects and keep you running longer, safer, and make for a faster return to the road.

If the shoe fits

Footwear very much varies by sport or exercise. During pregnancy, shoe size can change due to multiple factors including swelling and ligamentous laxity (relaxin again!) These can cause the bones to spread and the arch to drop, giving the foot a slightly longer length.

When it comes to what to wear when, here are my recommendations:

Yoga: Go barefoot! Pregnancy can cause balance and equilibrium changes and challenges due to both increase in body mass and laxity in the inner ear bones that give your body perception of where you are in space (hence, why some pregnant people get vertigo.) Nerves in your skin and joints communicate balance information to your brain, so having close contact with the floor or mat gives your body the best input and helps strengthen your foot and ankle muscles. Doing active barefoot yoga can help maintain balance as well as deep foot muscle strength, which supports the arches of your feet.

 Walking or running: Sneakers, of course. If you're already a runner, you likely have some kicks you love to take a ride in. Watch your foot size, as with the aforementioned hormone changes and added weight, your arch can drop, your foot can splay, and size can increase by length and/or width. The foam at the bottom of a shoe is designed to cushion you from ground impact, so something to look for in a shoe is good shock absorption.

 Hiking or uneven terrain: It's all about the ankle support with hiking or uneven terrain, so I recommend making sure you have good boots to support you. Relaxin creates more stretch to your ligaments and tendons, and your center of mass is changing with your bump so your balance can be off. A shoe that supports your ankles can help to prevent a sprain or fall.

CHAPTER 5:

The Stretches

Even for our less flexible friends.

Don't skip the stretching!

Stretching feels good and helps optimize the length of your muscles, decrease spasms and tension, and helps the position of your body and joints to facilitate labor for a smoother birth.

It's also a great way to implement deep breathing. Remember, stretching should be gentle—not painful. If you're normally pretty bendy, keep your stretches in a safe range to protect your joints.

Try doing each stretch three times for 30 seconds.

Here are my top six stretches that help your pelvis, inner core, and pelvic floor stay relaxed (but engaged) during your pregnancy, as well as open your pelvic floor muscles for delivery. These are easy stretches to do at home without a lot of equipment. All you need: some relaxing tunes, a yoga mat, two rolled blankets or yoga blocks, and a pillow or bolster for added support during your second and third trimesters.

It's important to note that relaxed does **not** equate weak. A normal pelvic floor muscle has *normal* tone, meaning it can contract and develop strength when it needs to. That also means that while in a "resting" state, it can hold your pelvic organs in place, as well as elongate and relax when it needs to, for sex and a vaginal birth.

Stretch 1: Deep Squat

This move stretches and releases your pelvic floor muscles and inner thigh muscles all at once.

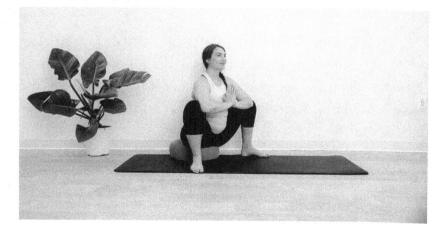

1. From standing, exhale and come down to a low, relaxed squat position, and visualize widening or separating your sit bones from each other.
2. Breathe deeply. With each breath in, visualize widening your sit bones like a flower blooming open, making way for safe passage for your baby. Stay here for 30-90 seconds, or for however long is comfortable.

Check in with your body: You can hold onto a bar or railing, lean backwards against the wall, put a rolled towel under your knees for support, or place a yoga block under your sit bones to modify this stretch and make it work better for your body. Not familiar with your sit bones? While sitting, reach your hand under the fleshy part of your butt cheek and feel the bony prominence that you sit on. Those are your "sit bones." No two bodies are the same, so modify to do what feels right for yours. None of the stretches should be painful or uncomfortable beyond an "I feel tight here" sensation.

Stretch 2: Happy Baby

This is another one of my favorite ways to lengthen and open your pelvic floor muscles and allow the release of your inner thigh muscles. The happy baby stretch is a great alternative to the deep squat stretch if that position doesn't feel right for your body at this time.

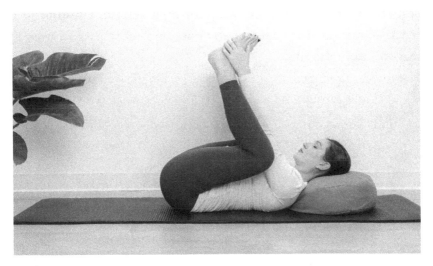

1. Come softly to the ground and lie on your back, slightly propped up with a pillow if you are in your second or third trimester and bring your legs wide.
2. Hold the outside edges of your feet with your legs perpendicular to the ground and visualize widening or separating your sit bones from each other. Breathe deeply. Remain here for 30-90 seconds, or for however long is comfortable.

Check in with your body: Finding it too tough to lay on the floor? Scoot your bottom toward a wall and put your feet along the wall in a gentle, wide V-shape, then try to relax into the pose. As with any of these exercises, if you ever feel flushed, dizzy, nauseous, or short of breath, change positions.

Stretch 3: Supported Butterfly

This move stretches and elongates the inner thigh muscles that begin at the pubic bone, allowing for their release. Use this as a gentle transition from happy baby pose to a more passive stretch that you can relax into.

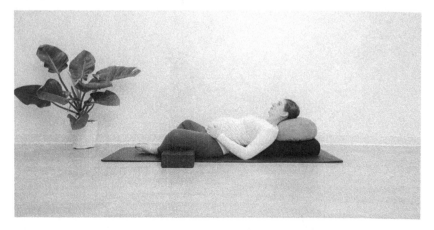

1. Lay slightly propped on a pillow so as to not be completely flat on your back. Bring together the soles of your feet while keeping your knees bent and splayed outwards.

2. Place a yoga block, pillow, or rolled blanket under each knee so that you feel a gentle but supported stretch. You can stay here for 30-90 seconds, or what is comfortable.

3. During this stretch, close your eyes and mindfully practice some alternate nostril breathing: inhale slowly through your left nostril and exhale back out through your right, alternating between left and right nostril every other breath. Traditionally in yoga practice, you would use your thumb to close the nostril you are not breathing through, so you can choose whichever method speaks to you. Alternate nostril breathing is meditative and relaxing; it's also another tool in your toolbox for pain management during labor and delivery.

Check in with your body: Need a modification? Perform this stretch upright: relax against a wall, and bring bent knees apart, splayed side to side, supported on a yoga block or rolled blanket for a gentle stretch. This stretch can also be performed laying down with your legs supported on the wall. Choose what feels best for you that day!

Stretch 4: The Figure 4

It's so important to stretch your piriformis, or deep hip rotator muscle, which is part of your deepest layer of pelvic floor muscles. This pose does just that.

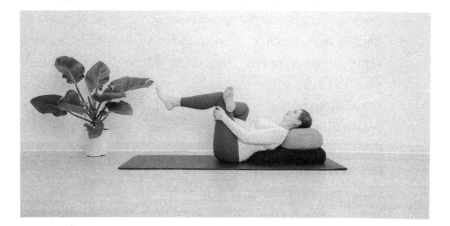

1. Lay slightly propped on a pillow so as to not be completely flat on your back and stretch your legs straight out. Cross one leg over the other, with the knee pointing out, like the shape of a number 4.

2. Lace your hands behind the hamstrings and thighs of your straightened bottom leg and gently draw your leg in toward your body by bending the straightened knee. You should feel this gentle stretch in your back pocket. Hold this position for 30 seconds 3 times for an optimal stretch. Repeat on the opposite side.

Check in with your body: Having trouble? You can also do this sitting on an exercise ball or in a chair, crossing one leg over the other like a number 4, and gently lean forward. Never force your body into a stretch it isn't comfortable with. As your baby grows and your belly gets bigger you won't be able to go as far—that's normal!

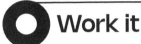

Work it

This is a great exercise to easily implement into your workday. If you are sitting at length for a call or meeting, cross one leg over the other in the number 4 position and lean gently forward until you feel a stretch in your back pocket. Peppering in stretches throughout the day helps both your mind and body to take a 30-second break to regroup and recharge.

Stretch 5: Cat/Cow

This pose helps with abdominal and pelvic floor muscle control as well as relaxation, offers gentle movement of your spine and pelvis, and helps better position the baby into the pelvis.

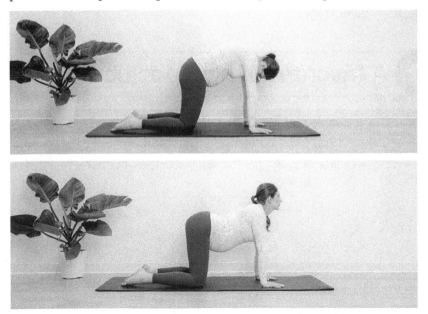

1. Come to the ground on all fours, either with flat hands or on fists if your wrists are sensitive.
2. With a gentle inhale, arch your back and look up gently, while bringing your belly lower. Think of a cow whose belly hangs low while their gaze looks outward and up. Stay within your comfortable range, trusting your body.
3. On your exhale, gaze downward and stretch your whole spine up toward the ceiling, focusing on your middle spine between your shoulder blades., Think of an angry cat, arching its back.
4. Alternate between these movements gently, at the pace of your own breath for 10 repetitions.

Check in with your body: As you enter your third trimester, cow pose may no longer feel right for you. If so, go into cat pose and then back to neutral or find a rhythm that feels good to you. Need a break? Widen your knees and ankles and drop into child's pose—the next stretch!

● A favorite birthing position

Many people find laboring or birthing on their hands and knees (quadruped) to be a comfortable alternative to laying on your back or standing. So, get familiar with how your body feels here!

Stretch 6: Child's Pose

This pose, which stretches and elongates your spinal muscles, back, and shoulder muscles, is a great pose to sink into while easing into breath.

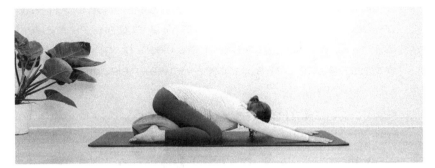

1. From cat/cow, widen your knees and bring your ankles out toward the edges of your mat. Then, drop your bottom between your ankles and your belly between your knees. Only come as low as you feel comfortable—listen to your body.

2. Draw your upper body down, arms wide, feeling a long stretch along your back. Let your belly rest gently between your knees. Stay here anywhere from 30 seconds to three minutes.

3. Play with widening your knees or ankles or whatever feels right to you in each trimester.

Check in with your body: Change things up! Bias your arms to one side to create a long, side-body stretch. For added support, add a bolster or yoga block under your sit bones.

⬤ Let in the light

Consider this: lighting a candle can help set the tone for relaxation. When you do this at a certain time each day, it signals to the body that it's time to slow down. During pregnancy (and anytime!), look for candles that are clean-burning, non-toxic, and free of artificial fragrances—or use an electric version.

Add this too: Breathwork

Alongside stretching, meditation, or yoga, breathwork is a great way to relax your body during pregnancy, while engaging your abdominal and pelvic muscles. The diaphragm, which sits under your ribs, works together with the pelvic floor muscles. When you inhale with a deep belly breath, the pelvic floor elongates and opens. When you exhale, the diaphragm draws upward and creates a pressure-driven pull upward in the abdomen that helps the pelvic floor to contract upwards. Essentially, breathwork helps the "dream team" of core muscles work together, even igniting a contraction of your deep abdominals at the end of the exhalation.

Relaxation or opening of your pelvic floor muscles is crucial for vaginal delivery. Breathwork paired with visualization also helps to control your physical body in response to discomfort or pain.

Try this: Find a comfortable, supported position while seated or lying down, and close your eyes. Place your hands on your heart space or on your growing belly. Then, visualize the wave:

You are on a remote beach sitting at the water's edge, feeling the warmth of the sand on your body, and the coolness of the sea lapping at your feet.

Your baby is warm and nurtured inside of you; you are kept cool by the breeze.

As the waves of contractions come, see these ocean waves rolling in, then breaking to foam, and releasing back to the sea.

Find your breath, inhale, filling your belly, elongating your pelvic floor. Feel the wave recede to the ocean.

Exhale, allow your baby to tuck in towards your spine, and your pelvic floor quietly contracts. Feel the wave gently roll onto the shore.

Repeat with your breath, feeling the opening and releasing as the wave returns to the ocean, followed by the rhythmic closing as the wave crashes to the shore.

Your baby is warm, thriving, and waiting to meet you.

You are cool, supported, and waiting to meet your baby.

Find your breath, inhale, filling your belly, elongating your pelvic floor. Feel the wave recede to the ocean.

Exhale, allow your baby to tuck in towards your spine, your pelvic floor quietly contracts. Feel the wave gently roll onto the shore.

The waves continue to gently crash, reminding you: you are safe, your baby is safe.

CHAPTER 6:

Sex, Sleep & Other Vitals

What your mama never told you about pregnancy

'd be remiss if I didn't discuss sleep and sex, as your relationship with both may go through some major changes during pregnancy—but don't worry! Not forever. I'll also touch on perineal massage, which can help prevent severe tearing during delivery... and how to ensure painless poops. You know, the fun stuff.

Seeking Sleep

You desperately need it, but sometimes it can be *so* difficult. Between the changes in your physical shape making it hard to find a comfortable position, the heat your pregnant body creates at night, and an anxious mind worrying about all of these changes, insomnia is hardly uncommon during pregnancy. Add in restless leg syndrome or heartburn and it's a wonder how anyone gets any shuteye. However, sleep is still super important—it's crucial for your body to recharge, recover, and rest.

Often, the most comfortable sleep position for many pregnant people is on their side—side-sleeping. When you lie on your back,

71

pressure from the growing placenta and baby can push down on your inferior vena cava, the large vein that brings all of your body's returning blood flow from the lower part of your body back to your heart. Compression of this large vein can cause hypotension (lowered blood pressure) leaving one feeling woozy, weak, and/or nauseated. Sleeping on your side is also best for your lower back.

If you're a back sleeper, talk to your OB/GYN about the risks to you and your baby from sleeping in this position and to find a solution. There is growing research that indicates any position is safe, but while that research is being processed by ACOG, stick to your side or confer with your doctor.

Pillows and props are the key—find one that works for you. You can use multiple pillows as different props, or one larger body pillow. Features to look for: versatility, cooling, and packable.

The 5 Sleep Hacks Every Pregnant Person Needs to Know:

1. **Make your nest:** While laying on your side, place one pillow between your knees and another between your ankles to create an even plane between your hip, knee, and ankle joints. The pillows should be oriented parallel in an ideal situation. As your bump grows, place a small pillow under your belly on the side for added support. Also try placing a pillow under your upper arm to reduce chest tightness and protect your posture.

2. **Bedtime routine:** Create a calming nightly routine, taking time each night to unwind your body slowly. Whether that includes lighting a candle, reading a book, or taking a relaxing bath with some lavender, find a way to unwind that speaks to you. Turn off any blue light producing electronics like phones, tablets, and laptops while you wind down!

3. **Hydrate well before bedtime:** Being hydrated in pregnancy is very important but try to get the H2O in well throughout the day and stop drinking fluids an hour before bed. This helps prevent unnecessary trips to the bathroom to urinate throughout the night.

4. **Set up a mindfulness practice:** Busy brain chatter makes sleep even more challenging. Try journaling, a meditation app, or doing stretches and breathwork in the evenings to help prepare your body for sleep.

5. **Make time for exercise:** Moderate aerobic activity has been widely demonstrated through research to improve the amount of deep sleep you get, although the exact reason why has yet to be revealed.

Sex During Pregnancy

Without a doubt, sex and pleasure can be different—and feel different—for every pregnant person. It can also change throughout pregnancy or gestation. "Sex" encompasses a wide range of play, whether that's using a sex toy, a finger, a penis, oral sex, or intimacy. Sex, pleasure, and intimacy are spectrums no longer boxed in by outdated cultural and societal standards: sex and intimacy are defined by you and your relationship.

During pregnancy, some people have heightened levels of arousal and/or increased sensitivity to touch, especially at nipples and erogenous zones. Increased blood flow to the vulva, breasts, and pelvic organs can increase sensitivity and contribute to increased arousal, as can the surge of hormones your body is experiencing. The rise in estrogen and progesterone are to blame for this one!

It is not uncommon to have sexual dreams while pregnant or feel hornier than you've ever been before! This is also a fun time to play and explore. Arousal and sex increase blood flow to the pelvic organs, pelvic floor tissues, and muscles, all good things during pregnancy. Penetrative sex allows pelvic floor tissues to stretch and adapt, as well as contract with orgasm and control of penetration, which is exercising these muscles.

However, others may experience lowered levels of arousal or interest in sex. Morning sickness, fatigue, and discomfort of a growing body can all be deterrents to sex. Some pregnant people (or their partners) worry about the risks to the fetus or baby while having sex—discuss these concerns with your doctor or birth provider. As always, consult your birth or medical care team if you have any medical concerns, prior to engaging in sexual activities.

Some people feel wildly sexy while pregnant, with hormones surging and sexual drive rocketing, while others feel sluggish, with breast tenderness or a total lack of libido. These are all normal responses and bodily adaptations, and they can change throughout pregnancy. So, tune in and do what feels right for you.

If you are cleared for vaginal penetration by your doctor/ midwife, use a pregnancy-safe, paraben-free, glycerin-free lubricant and get busy! You may need to change your position, or use extra support, like pillows, during sex. Masturbation is also a great option for some fun, stress-reducing self-care. Either way, arousal and orgasms help draw good blood flow to the pelvis, release happy hormones and strengthen the pelvic floor.

Controlling depth: This is a complaint from many pregnant people: they feel like they can't tolerate the same amount of depth as before. This is where changing positions (pregnant person on top) or using a product such as the OhNut, which allows for the feel of depth for both partners but acts as a bumper or guard against it, are great options.

A note on pain: Sex shouldn't be painful—if it is, stop and consult your OB, midwife, or pelvic physical therapist. Painful sex or orgasm could mean that you need to change the position you are in, or it could mean tight or spasmed muscles, vaginal dryness, anxiety. In some cases, it could mean you have a genital or pelvic infection. If you are experiencing pain during sex at all, reach out for help.

Sex therapy: Sex therapists are specially trained and certified mental health therapists that go through an additional rigorous education and certification process to work with clients that have sexual trauma, sexual concerns, partner concerns, need help with intimacy, pleasure, orgasm, sex drive, and so forth. Whether this is a pregnancy issue, something that has been brewing for some time, or starts postpartum, I always like to highlight this helpful resource for my clients.

Sex Positions to Consider

This widely varies based on the kind of sex you enjoy and the anatomy, or toy play, of the person(s) you are enjoying it with. Positions you would normally engage in are fine during pregnancy, but what might feel comfortable during your first trimester might not the third. If you feel any pain or discomfort, switch!

Side-lying: Consider laying on your side with a pillow under your top knee, which is flexed slightly higher than your bottom knee, to allow your partner to penetrate from behind. This position is great for off weighting the pressure of the belly, being able to relax into the experience, and is also a great position if you are experiencing SPD, or hip or low back pain. For some people that have experienced trauma or a sexual experience without their consent, a partner coming from behind may feel triggering. I encourage you to find a consensual position that feels comfortable for you.

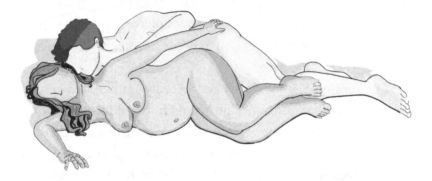

Quadruped (aka doggy style): Rest on all fours, even putting your forearms and head down on the bed or surface to off-weight more of the belly. Leaning against a wall or in the shower, or having your partner sit on a chair and face away, is also an option during pregnancy to have more control and variety. If you want to control the depth and speed of penetration while engaging your pelvic floor muscles well, you can also squat on top. However, this position is less ideal if you have deep hip pain or SPD during pregnancy.

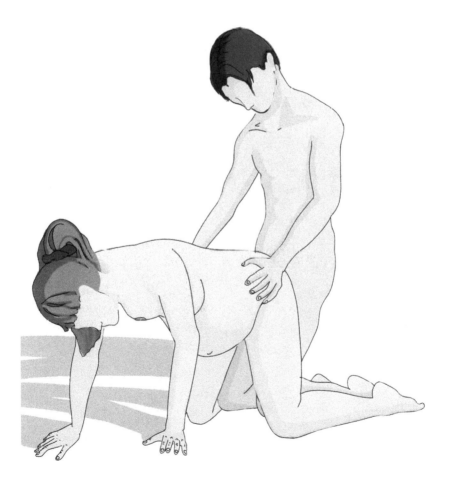

Semi-reclined: Think of this as missionary with a boost. Bonus? You can do this at the edge of a bed or couch and your partner can stand.

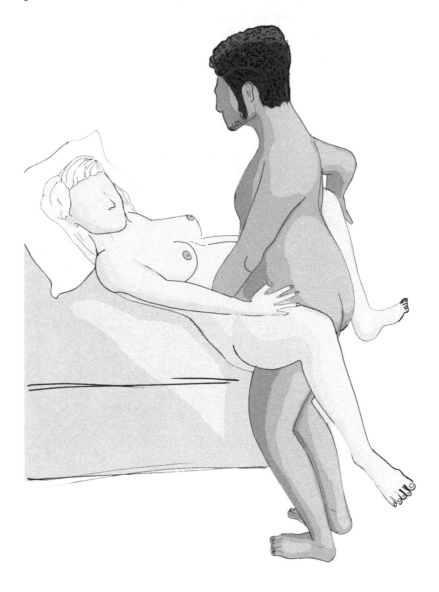

Oral sex: Relax and lay supported or semi-reclined, seated, or standing against a wall—or even sitting on your birth ball! There are many positions to enjoy this experience in.

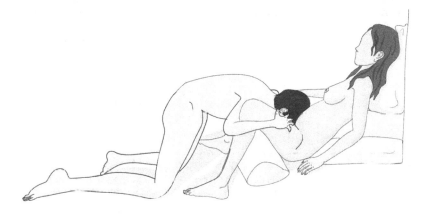

The Wide World of Lubes

The world of lubricants is ever changing and advancing for our benefit: so, find one that you like! Always look for lubricants that are FDA-approved; fragrance-, paraben- and glycerin-free; many options are now gluten-free and vegan as well. As with any new skincare product, always test a small amount on your wrist in advance to ensure you don't have a negative reaction. Here are some of the different lubricant varieties and their best uses:

TYPE	USES	NOTES
Water-based lubricants	Penetration, intercourse, toy play, or perineal massage.	Can be used with toys and condoms—won't break down either condoms or toys.
Oil-based lubricants	Intercourse, massage, or perineal massage.	Coconut oil should not be used for some people with tree-nut sensitivities or who have a history of repeat vaginal infections. Oil formulas break down condoms and cannot be used with some toys.
Aloe-based lubricants	Penetration, intercourse, toy play, or perineal massage.	Can be used with toys and condoms—won't break down either; however, aloe-based lubricants are not as commonly found.
Silicone-based lubricants	Penetration, intercourse, or perineal massage. Silicone-based lubricants are better for shower/water or anal play because silicone does not evaporate. As a result, it remains lubricating longer.	Cannot be used with silicone-based sex toys because silicone on silicone causes a breakdown in materials. However, since they do not contain any water (a requirement for bacteria), silicone-based lubricants do not require preservatives and are pH neutral for the vagina.

All About Poop: Keep the BMs Movin'!

Regular elimination is super important for about a zillion reasons, one of which is removing excess hormones and waste products from the body. I probably don't have to tell you that constipation is not uncommon during pregnancy as your abdominal organs are more tightly compacted due to your growing baby, hormonal changes, as well as shifts in your normal activity and exercise—all of which may slow things down.

The pregnancy hormone progesterone helps to relax smooth muscle, which is the type of muscle that surrounds your intestine and helps things to move along. As this hormone increases, bowels can slow down in motility. Maintaining a fiber-rich diet, regular hydration, and consistent activity can all aid in movement. The placenta releases gastrin, which can cause an increase in gastric acidity. Smooth muscle relaxation around the sphincters in your esophagus, as well as the increased pressure upward on the diaphragm, can contribute to reflux. Your birth provider or medical doctor can help you safely address these concerns or refer you to a gastroenterologist if they become more severe.

Here's where my experience as a pelvic physical therapist comes in: using a stool under your feet while you poop can help prevent straining, which can lead to unwanted hemorrhoids or pelvic floor changes. Ideally, you want a slight "squat" position, with your knees above the level of your hips. Stool height will vary depending upon your toilet height. But your goal is to have at least one bowel movement daily—otherwise, transit time can be too long, and stool becomes harder and more difficult to pass.

Your pelvic floor muscles provide support to your rectum, placing it at an optimal angle to prevent stool from just, well... sliding out. Although it may feel like pushing and straining can help you eliminate, it actually tightens these muscles, creating a smaller opening which makes stool even harder to pass. Proper positioning while you poop paired with open-mouthed breathing and the tips below can help keep you regular.

6 Easy Ways to Keep Stool Moving

1. **Get in position**: Use a low stool under your feet to prop your knees up higher than your hips, like a seated squat. This helps open the pelvic floor and relaxes your muscles, allowing poop to move along. Tip: This is also a comfortable laboring position, and many people find laboring on the toilet their favorite position

2. **Drink up:** Staying well-hydrated is key to smooth elimination.

3. **Fill up on fiber:** Implement soft fibers like fruit, pears and berries into your diet, or non-sugar fibers like psyllium husk if you are watching sugar levels. Seek out a midwife or a nutritionist that specializes in prenatal care if you have dietary needs or concerns, gestational diabetes, or continue to struggle.

4. **Stop the rush:** It's important to listen to your body's cues. Try to recognize your natural urge to eliminate and set aside enough time to do so where you're not overly stressed. The bowels like routine!

5. **Open your mouth:** Sounds strange, but open mouth = open orifices. Relax, don't bear down or hold your breath, and breathe with an open mouth during a bowel movement.

6. **Get moving:** Those with more sedentary lifestyles are more likely to experience constipation. Movement can literally help move things along.

The name of the game? Don't strain. If you're struggling to have regular bowel movements, be sure to reach out to your OB, midwife, pelvic floor physical therapist, nutritionist, or registered dietitian to talk about options.

Perineal Massage

The perineum is the area of tissue between the vaginal opening and the anus. This area is where the skin, fascia, soft tissues, and muscles of the superficial (first layer of pelvic floor muscles) layer, as well as anal sphincters, connect centrally at the perineal body. The perineum and perineal body are critical to pelvic floor function. The perineum also creates the boundaries for the vagina and the anus.

Probably the number one question I get asked from pregnant clients is, "How do I avoid tearing during birth?" There are a thousand different scenarios and contributors to tearing or other birth injuries. Your anatomy, the size/anatomy of your baby, position of birth, previous injuries, length of labor/delivery, breath mechanics, pelvic floor strength and length, tissue quality, interventions such as forceps or the vacuum, and sometimes, luck. Research continues to grow in this area, but currently points to perineal massage as a way to lessen the risk of significant (grade 3 or 4) tear during birth and the risk of an episiotomy.

Perineal Massage in the Third Trimester

Perineal massage is a way to become intimate with your vulvo-vaginal area during pregnancy, and crucially, it helps you understand what is normal versus not postpartum. Taking a hand mirror and looking at your vulvar tissues or using fingers to explore your anatomy and perform perineal massage are important ways to familiarize yourself with your before—or baseline. Knowing the "before" helps you to determine the differences, or your specific needs, postpartum.

All this said, some people just aren't comfortable doing perineal massage. The good thing is, you get to choose if this is a tool you would like to utilize in your pregnancy toolbox!

Currently, we have no solid, evidence-based research to indicate this is a "make it or break it" act to perform during pregnancy. What we do know is that it does help elongate tissues and muscles, increase blood flow to the area, and assist with muscle and tissue relaxation in areas that will need to accommodate for stretch. The choice for perineal massage is ultimately up to you.

How to Perform Perineal Massage

Perineal massage is best utilized during the third trimester, at week 34 and beyond. You can perform perineal massage solo, or have your partner perform it for you.

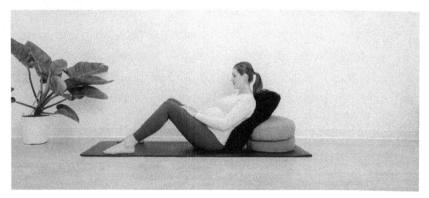

Begin by laying down in a comfortable position. This could mean your back and head are slightly inclined or propped up with pillows, or it could mean laying on your side with a pillow between your knees. What is important is that your legs are supported and relaxed, and your hand can access your vaginal opening comfortably. Have your knees bent and angled up, but relaxed open over a pillow. This position allows your butt, leg, and pelvic floor muscles to relax, while allowing you to comfortably reach your perineum. As an alternative, many people find doing this after a warm bath helps ensure they're super comfortable and blissed out.

The How-To:
1. Use clean hands and a lubricant you've chosen works best for you given my recommendations on page 80
2. Gently insert your thumb (or if doing this with a partner, their index finger) approximately one or two knuckles deep into the vagina. Apply pressure down toward your feet or down and back towards your anorectal area.
3. In a sweeping or windshield wiper motion, sweep back and forth along the perineum tissue from left to right and right to left. Imagine that you are sliding your thumb from hip to hip while lightly pulling downward. Use only gentle force; this should not be painful or intense. Do this for 3-5 minutes nightly.

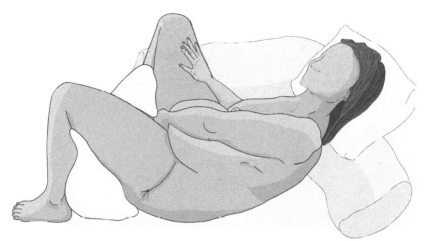

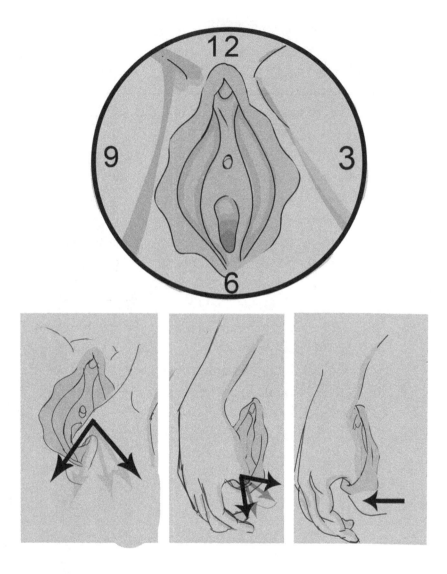

PART 3:
BIRTHING YOUR BABY

CHAPTER 7:

Laboring & Pushing

Push it real good

Prepping for Pushing:

By this point, you've done the bulk of the hard work: strengthened the muscles required for the endurance you'll need for labor, practiced various breathing techniques, and stretched literally everything. Look at you!

But in order to really thrive through the main event, you'll need to learn how to push. Ideal pushing involves knowing how to relax the body and the pelvic floor muscles—easier said than done when you're in the throes of labor. This is the primary reason why, toward the end of your pregnancy, I encourage using relaxation and pelvic-opening techniques rather than the hundreds of pelvic floor contractions that used to be the prescribed norm.

Pick Your Position

The first step in the pushing phase is to find a position to labor in that is not only comfortable for *your* body and where you are pushing (i.e., tub vs. bed), but one that helps to widen the pelvic outlet and utilizes gravity effectively to aid your muscles in pushing the baby out of your pelvis during birth.

Labor lasts different amounts of time for each individual. Birth plans and expectations, resources, and home birth versus hospital-based or birth center care can change or dictate certain parts of laboring. *Pelvic Prep School* does not provide the extensive information about different interventions, birth planning, or partner support that you may find with your birth provider, medical doctor, doula, or other birthing resources. Additionally, consulting your pelvic physical therapist for specific positional modifications based on your body can be exceptionally helpful.

For instance, if you have unresolved SPD or a history of tailbone pain, your choice of position may look different than another person's without that history. Depending on which stage of labor you're in, you may cycle through a few different positions. Here's where a well-trained birth partner or support person such as a doula can come in handy: they can guide you through the options.

Potential Birthing Positions

Below are options of many different birthing positions. Remember: no single position is best for everyone, and no single position will likely work for your entire labor or birth. I'm here to tell you that it's OK to move around as often as needed, with the assistance of your medical team, to positions that feel best and will be helpful in progressing your labor.

If you are limited from getting out of bed due to constant fetal monitoring, an epidural, or any other reason, I encourage you to ask your healthcare team for help in modifying positions. This could include using a peanut ball between your knees or guiding you to safe and comfortable positions to facilitate pelvic opening and perineal support.

Standing/squatting supported by partner, squat bar, or secured railing

- **Pros**: Squatting widens the diameter of the pelvic outlet, gives space for the tailbone and sacrum to extend out of the way, facilitates opening of the pelvic floor muscles, optimizes use of gravity, and feels like a natural position for a birthing person to sense the feeling of needing to deeply push. This position can be helpful if the baby is slow to descend.

- **Cons**: This position is not feasible with an epidural. It also requires a fair amount of leg and core strength. However, if the baby is descending too quickly, move in and out of this position and ask for perineal support.

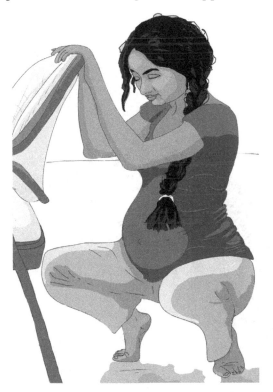

Kneeling upright or using a birthing seat or birth ball

- **Pros**: Kneeling or using a birthing seat/ball also widens the pelvic outlet and gives space for the tailbone to extend out of the way. It requires less leg strength and endurance than standing/squatting, and it's good for people who may have pain with weightbearing through their arms. In this position you'll also be able to go into a half-kneeling stance, with one knee up and one leg on the ground, which may help with the descent of the baby, depending on positioning.
- **Cons**: This position is not feasible with an epidural. It's also not ideal for people with pre-existing spinal instabilities or those who experience any discomfort on their knees.

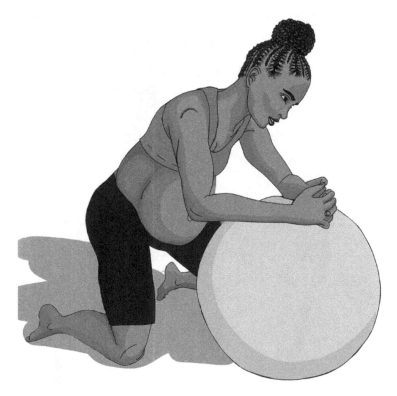

Traditional: Semi-reclined
(laying on your back with legs up)

- **Pros**: The traditional birth position allows for epidural administration, and the pregnant person can have help changing hip positions when needed for comfort or due to previous injuries. It's often preferred in hospitals as it allows providers easy access. It's also a great position for using a hand mirror to watch the baby descend and motivate pushing.

- **Cons**: Laying on your back places weight on the sacrum and tailbone, does not allow as much room for the tailbone to extend or joints to move, and does not let gravity assist in delivery. It's not ideal for people who are experiencing back labor pain or tailbone pain.

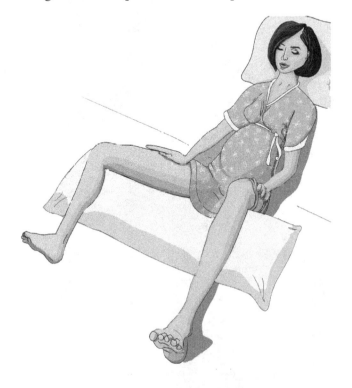

Side–lying (use of birthing peanut or partner)

- **Pros**: Side-lying allows for an epidural, allows for rest of the whole body between contractions, takes pressure off of the sacrum and tailbone, and widens the pelvic outlet if legs are positioned with knees in and ankles out, like being pigeon-toed. It also allows the tailbone to extend out of the way and gives the perineum time to elongate. It's good for people with pre-existing back conditions.
- **Cons**: This position may be uncomfortable if you have a history of hip pain. It's also anti-gravity, so this position does not assist with descent of the baby.

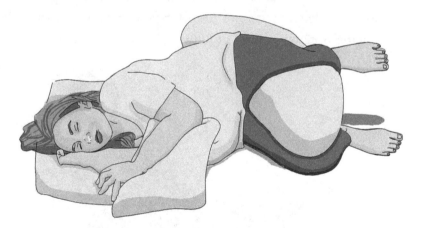

Quadruped (on hands and knees)

- **Pros**: Birthing on your hands and knees widens the pelvic outlet, gives space for the tailbone to extend out of the way, facilitates opening of the pelvic floor muscles, and may be restful between contractions (try bending your head to your elbows). This is a good position for support persons to give counter pressure and massage, and it allows gravity to help with the descent of the baby. It's also fine for people with pre-existing back conditions.
- **Cons**: This position is not feasible with an epidural and may not be ideal for people who have pain bearing weight through their arms. It also may make some people feel too vulnerable.

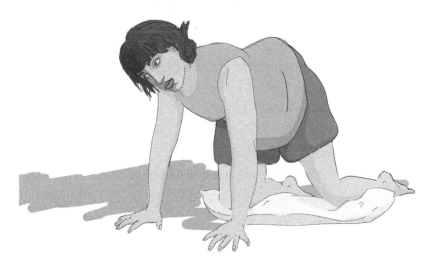

Ready to Push? Yes, You Are!

Here's the key—don't forget to breathe! Traditionally, a pushing method known as "blocked inhalation" was the gold standard, where birthing people would inhale, and then hold their breath, contract their abdominals down, and push down forcefully. But here's the problem with that: holding your breath, known as valsalva, will increase tension in your body, ratchet up resistance in the pelvic floor, and cause adverse effects on your cardiovascular system.

Imagine holding your breath and bearing down as hard as you can (imagine, don't actually do this!) All of this pressure not only can make you see stars but think about the pressure this is creating on your pelvic organs and tissues as well the abdominal stuff above that gets squashed down. This increase in pressure may be why many people report hemorrhoids, prolapse, or other pressure-related injuries post-pushing.

It's important to recognize there are several methods taught for pushing, and most rely on knowledge of the anatomy, pressure systems in the body, biomechanics, plus practitioner experience and low-level evidence. (High-quality evidence-based practice remains scarce in the field of birth delivery.) To reduce the downward impact on the pelvic organs and support important pelvic floor function, here's the method I prefer based on both training and experience:

- THE PELVIC PREP SCHOOL PUSHING PRACTICE
  1. Start in a supported reclined position, like sitting in bed while leaning back on some pillows.
  2. Take a moment to center yourself in your body: remind yourself that you are safe, your baby is safe, and your body inherently knows what to do.

3. Take in a slow, steady, deep breath through your nose or mouth (this will vary on comfort during labor)

4. Gently tense the abdomen, contract through the abdominal wall, and slowly breathe out, exhaling with a "HAAA" sound while maintaining the abdominal pressure. Maintain as much relaxation as you can in your legs and pelvic floor area.

5. Exhale for 5-7 counts as you relax the pelvic floor and pelvic floor muscles.

6. Repeat these steps ten times, 2-3 times per day.

Good to Know:

Once you feel like you've got this down, practice in different positions. This practice can be used in many positions, whether you are water birthing, squatting, laying down, using medication or birthing unmedicated. Notice where you feel most comfortable—which may change during true labor—but also be mindful of your pelvic floor muscles and how they feel in each position.

Because every body is different and we all have varying levels of familiarity with what feels "right" when we move or use different parts of our bodies, it can be beneficial to many pregnant persons to make this a point of conversation with their birthing resources, whether it be doula, pelvic floor physical therapist, birth provider, medical provider, or another experienced individual in this field. The most important thing is to learn how to properly tense your abdomen and relax your pelvic floor.

During active birth, focus on "letting go" of your pelvic floor and breathing with light panting or groans to encourage relaxation of your pelvic floor. Keeping your throat open as much as possible helps to maintain an opening through your pelvic floor and helps to prevent the valsalva (breath hold and bracing) I mentioned earlier. Align this practice with other resources shared by your birth provider, such as patterned-breathing, meditative birth practices, or training. Find what feels best for your body but know that can change—and that is OK!

CHAPTER 8:

Delivery & Recovery

So you never have to say, "Why didn't anyone tell me this part?"

Pregnancy and birth are often the most intensely physical transformation of a person's life—and that shouldn't be minimized. Regardless of your method of birth, the preparation of your pelvic floor and abdominal muscles is integral to your post-birth recovery. This chapter dives into the birth, delivery, and recovery processes for both vaginal and C-section births.

I Repeat: All Birth is Natural

Many individuals go into their birth experience with the goal of a vaginal birth. But just as many others choose a cesarean section birth (C-section) or have a medical or social history that indicates a C-section is the safer option. It's my view that regardless of the way your baby enters the world, it is natural. Medicated, unmedicated, vaginal, C-section, multiples, all are natural. My goal is to help you anticipate your pelvic floor's needs and prepare your pelvis and body for any outcome.

Vaginal Birth

A vaginal birth can occur at home, in a birthing center, or a hospital-based setting. After a vaginal birth and delivery of the placenta, you can expect some level of swelling in your perineal and vaginal area, and you may have some pain or discomfort. Always ask: that's what the wonderful nurses and doctors of the L&D ward are there for, or your midwife in aftercare. They understand this is a totally new experience for (most of) you. I cannot stress enough: you know your body better than anyone else and will be your own #1 advocate if something does not feel right to you.

Bleeding, or lochia, will begin from the place where your placenta was attached to the inside of your uterus—a wound the size of an average dinner plate. Pay close attention to this bleeding, monitoring it for clots and color, and communicate with your healthcare team about what you're seeing. You may see lochia for up to six weeks post-birth as your uterus begins to contract and retract to its approximate original size and location in your body.

Cesarean Section Birth

A cesarean section birth involves an incision through the lower abdominal skin, fat tissues, connective tissues, and fascia. Then, the lower abdominals are separated—not cut into—before an incision to the thick, muscular uterine wall. Many people make the mistake of believing that inner core strength and stability is compromised due to muscular incisions, when actually, it's all physics!

Think about a bridge: it has several different types of materials to hold it up—rebar, concrete, more flexible things that can give some bend and give for motion. In this case, you have fascia (a type of connective tissue), muscles, scar tissue. When we cause some damage, dysfunction, or realign one of those materials, things just don't work exactly like they should. This causes some instability in the core or a change in some of the ways your body subtly moves.

Add that you may have had pain and/or atrophy of some of your abdominal muscles due to disuse post C-section, and your core might need a serious pep talk postpartum. This is a great reason to strengthen your inner core area during pregnancy. Following a C-section, you'll be limited in your mobility immediately postpartum, and your healing time may be lengthened as opposed to a vaginal delivery.

Similar to a vaginal birth, C-section births can also result in incontinence, scar tissue, or pelvic pain. However, regardless of method of birth, parents have wonderful birth outcomes, and if concerns arise, they can be addressed through a professional care team with a thorough understanding of healing.

Other Birth Interventions

Other birth interventions that are used sparingly and selectively to expedite birth under extreme circumstances are episiotomies, forceps, and vacuums. An episiotomy is often a laceration performed to expedite fetal expulsion (aka to get the baby out). Forceps delivery is when forceps, or a medical grade spatula, are placed intravaginally and around the fetus to aid in delivery, while a vacuum uses pressure to aid in expediting the birth. These birth interventions can cause tears or lacerations in the perineal and/or pelvic floor tissues.

Literature and obstetric guidelines promote informed consent to the birthing person, when able, and/or their medical proxy. Informed consent is when a procedure, its full risks, and benefits are explained in detail so the person receiving the procedure can make an educated decision prior to giving consent. Take time in your prenatal appointments to discuss your practice's use of these techniques, have an open dialogue with your provider and your expectations and needs, and ask questions.

Birth Pain Management and Support

Epidurals

An epidural procedure is when medication is given via an anesthesiologist to numb the area between the belly button and mid to upper legs so that during a long labor you can rest, have pain relief, but also be awake, alert, and feel pressure to push during active birthing when it is time. Your doula, birth partner, or care team can aid in assisting you to move positions from back to on your side and so forth, but you cannot be up and walking once or out of bed once you have an epidural.

Doulas

Many people opt for labor support in the form of a doula to mitigate pain, aid in the informed consent process, and prolong the timeframe between going into labor and entering the hospital by laboring at home. A doula is a form of birth support—educational, physical and emotional—from a trained professional who aids the birthing person either prenatally, during birth, or postpartum.

A doula is not a medical professional but has completed certifications and training. They can provide support such as position changes, breath work, labor tools such as birthing balls, etc. to assist in pain relief and comfort measures during birth. Many hospitals now offer free doula support during labor and birthing, or you can hire a doula to attend your birth.

One More Time for the People in the Back: All Birth is Natural!

I encourage my clients to consider all options because all birth is natural. What is right for one person and their medical history—whether it be trauma, prior birthing experiences, past medical history, pain tolerance, or just expectations for an emotionally and physically satisfying birth— there are many ways to labor and birth. Not all ways are right for all people. There's also the fact that emergencies happen. Flipped babies happen. The most important thing is to know that no matter what happens, you can heal on the other side of it.

Recovery from birth: Vaginal

The recovery from a vaginal birth can vary exceptionally. All the preparation you have done for your pelvis, pelvic floor muscles, and your changing body has already gone a long way!

Swelling will be addressed immediately postpartum—your provider will provide you with cooling methods, whether ice packs or cool towels, and recommend protocols specific to your care. Hospitals often provide extra ice packs to go upon request. Sometimes swelling can be quite significant, especially if you had any tearing, abrasions, or other interventions. Your medical care team can provide more insight on immediate swelling, however, understand that sometimes the swelling can "mask" other things that might be going on. For instance, some individuals don't report much incontinence until the swelling has actually gone down, they feel more pelvic pressure, or dropping of the pelvic floor, which is like the sensation of a tampon falling out.

If you aren't up for making DIY "padsicles" at home (frozen sanitary pads made at home with aloe and witch hazel) you can purchase postpartum underwear with pockets or gussets for adding ice packs to manage pain and swelling from both vaginal and C-section deliveries. Either way, cooling for short time periods can help.

Recovery from birth: Cesarean

When the entire abdominal canister (which includes your diaphragm, your pelvic floor, and your abdominals) is disrupted and altered, everything from your strength, coordination, and muscle recruitment to your endurance, breath, movement patterns, and pelvic floor health may be impacted. A C-section scar may affect how the components of this canister work together due to pain, scar tissue, and/or restrictions in your ability to move. It's a big deal.

Your provider will likely provide you with a brace or a stretchy, fabric corset to go around your waist to help support you as you move and to prevent over-activation of your muscles while they heal. But once healed, the goal is to learn to properly engage and activate your abdominal muscles to strengthen them—not to rely on a brace for long-term assistance.

During those first few weeks at home, it's vital to learn how to care for your infant and also aid your own recovery when movement is limited. Practicing gentle breathwork or adopting pain modification strategies (even what you used during labor!) are easy to do in tandem to caring for your newborn.

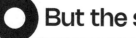

But the scar!

In the world of postpartum, you may be flooded with social media or internet information on what to do post c-section birth. One of these topics is performing massage on your scar with either your hands, or a tool, to promote it to fade, get thinner and not feel so "stuck." Professionally, we refer to this as scar release. Any scar release should only be performed once all wounds have closed, scabs have fallen off, and you have been cleared by your medical professional. Remember, many layers were disrupted, so we want each to have time to heal. Additionally, scar release should never be aggressive or cause bruising.

FAQs

I love a good FAQ section, and thought it'd be helpful to get a few of the post-birth basics covered here:

Q. What can I do in the first few days after birth?

A: Practice your diaphragmatic breathwork. You can begin this right away, and it is safe regardless of your method of birthing. Breathwork encourages your deep abdominals to engage at the end of the breath and will help your abdominal and pelvic floor muscles to begin coordinating and working together again. I also love using breathwork for pain management during C-section birth recovery—not to mention in the big picture, it helps you relax in moments of stress.

Q. When should I start pelvic floor exercises?

A. Immediately postpartum, some may tell you to begin performing pelvic floor contractions. My recommendation? Let your pelvic floor and vulvovaginal area take some time to heal and reduce swelling prior to making any decisions regarding pelvic floor strengthening. Typically, I encourage my clients to spend the first 2-4 weeks postpartum getting to know Baby, resting, healing, and transitioning to parenthood. Then they should make an appointment with a pelvic floor physical therapist, who can assess when—or whether—you should start doing pelvic floor contractions. Often, clients need medical clearance from their birth provider (OB/GYN, midwife, etc.) prior to seeing another provider.

Q. When should I see my doctor/reach out to a pelvic physical therapist?

A. If you have a relatively uneventful birth and are taking it easy, seeing your OB/midwife at 4-6 weeks postpartum is the standard. I recommend you form a relationship with a pelvic physical therapist prior to your child's birth (just a one-time visit is sufficient in many cases), then reach out after your baby is born for a postpartum assessment—after you've been cleared by your physician or midwife. Take that hand mirror and sneak a peek of the postpartum "you" down there.

I Know You Want to Know: What is Tearing— and How Can I Avoid It?

Tearing involves a literal tear in the perineal tissue or soft tissues of the vaginal area (and potentially the muscles that lie underneath it) during delivery. Tearing severity is based on the degree of tear and layers of muscles that are involved. An abrasion (commonly referred to as skid marks or tiny cuts that do not require suturing) may not require any stitches but is still a superficial injury of your tissues.

Tears are graded by your doctor or surgeon by depth, ranging from superficial to most deep, or extensive. First-degree tearing is the mildest, while fourth-degree tears are the most severe and extend to/through the anorectal area and all layers of the pelvic floor muscles.

A severe tear may initially impact movement, walking, sitting in certain positions, continence (urine, fecal, or gas) and pain levels. Severe tears are associated with increased pain and pelvic floor dysfunction, such as pain during sex upon insertion, with tampon use, or during exercise. However, it is important to note that each person's healing process, pain levels and tolerance, and tissue healing are different. To be clear: pain once closure of tissues and sutures have dissolved is **not** normal and should be addressed. Pain with sex, an exam, touch, an orgasm, with urination or defecation, or any kind of incontinence is not normal.

Some individuals have more significant tears without dysfunction afterwards, but many women with more extensive tearing will report pain at some point during their fourth trimester or postpartum period.

Treating a Tear

Pelvic physical therapists are trained to help with the treatment and reduction of scar tissue after a tear, whether from birthing or a birth intervention, as well as associated pain, continence, and other dysfunction. It's important to note, however, that there are short windows of time where scar treatment can be the most helpful in healing, which is why we prefer to see birthing parents soon after they're deemed ready by their birth practitioner. Scar tissue can also be treated long after delivery (even years after!), but it is more optimal to treat scars during their initial healing phase.

Tearing Prevention

Appropriate pushing techniques, relaxation and opening of the pelvic floor muscles, perineal support by your birth team during delivery, and positioning during birth can all reduce the incidence of tearing, although there are thus far no research-supported clinical guidelines to fully and completely prevent tearing. And while there is a lot of talk about preventing tearing by not having an epidural, so you can feel more and reposition, be on all fours, etc., there isn't any big, good, juicy clinical evidence in that either. And the reality is, for some people the epidural is a godsend!

Basically, there's no recipe for total avoidance of tearing. But I caution you against fearing it. The body has incredible resilience and methods of healing. I encourage you to discuss risks, interventions, and methods used by your birth practitioners to have a greater understanding of both the tearing and healing processes prior to birth.

Pain: What's Common, What's Not

Initially, with a vaginal birth, you should expect some discomfort, tenderness, and swelling. If there is severe pain, unusual discharge, odor, or anything that just feels "off" to you, you should call your doctor.

Pain that lasts beyond the first few weeks, including vaginal pain, vulvar pain, a feeling of downward pressure in your vagina, tailbone pain, perineal pain, vaginal tightness or feelings of restriction, or C-section scar tightness, discomfort, or pain, should also merit an appointment with a pelvic physical therapist.

Postpartum assessments should be the norm. A pelvic physical therapist can evaluate and assess your pelvic floor tissues and muscles and educate you on scar release, relaxation techniques for your pelvic floor and other appropriate tips and methods specific to you. There's no reason you should experience pelvic pain, incontinence, or other forms of discomfort if you don't have to.

If you learn one thing from this book, let it be understood that pain during sex or penetration is NOT NORMAL. That applies to when you're allowed to have sex again, typically after about six weeks postpartum. While it might be painful or uncomfortable the first time or first few times, I encourage you to speak to your birth team after you deliver regarding *any* pain you may be experiencing in your vulvovaginal area that is persistent.

Contrary to popular belief, incontinence (leaking urine, feces, or gas) is also NOT NORMAL, and can happen regardless of your method of birth or delivery. Leaking is easily addressed and goes well beyond pelvic floor contractions. But remember—leaking can sometimes be caused by overly tight muscles or scar tissue. Think before you kegel—and reach out to a pelvic physical therapist if you're unsure.

Myth Busting

It's a total myth that you should wait until you're finished having kids to address any pelvic pain or other concerns. Incontinence, prolapse, diastasis recti, scar tissue pain are all signs that something's either too weak, too tight, or not functioning properly. Just as you devoted time and energy into labor and delivery prep, it's equally important to devote time and energy into healing from the changes of pregnancy and birth.

For more personalized information on your own recovery journey, returning to exercise, and what's next after delivery, I highly recommend making an appointment with a pelvic floor physical therapist. I just can't help myself—after all, it's my job and my mission!

Fun fact: did you know pelvic floor physical therapy postpartum people is a standard offering in many European countries, Australia, and New Zealand?

PART 4:

RESOURCES & THE POSTPARTUM TRANSITION

CHAPTER 9:

Tools & Building Your Team

DRAFTING YOUR DREAM TEAM

t's true: birthing a human takes a village. There are many different options for support depending on your needs and desires. Doing all of these things or none of these things does not provide any guarantees in pregnancy, labor, or delivery, but each has its added benefits and advantages. Don't be overwhelmed by the length of this list: pick one or a few that resonate with you.

- **Pelvic physical therapist:** Evaluates and treats pelvic floor dysfunction, such as pain or incontinence, and prenatal or postpartum musculoskeletal issues, such as diastasis recti, low back pain, symphysis pubic pain, pelvic congestion, or hip pain.

- **Birth or postpartum doula:** Doulas are professionally trained to support a birthing person emotionally and physically during pregnancy, labor, and/or postpartum.

- **Lactation consultant:** Certified lactation consultants offer support both pre- and post-birth and throughout your breastfeeding journey by assisting in breastfeeding and pumping education.

- **Chiropractic care:** A doctor of chiropractic care specially trained in prenatal and postpartum care may provide pain relief and help with optimal labor positioning.
- **Childbirth educator:** Birth classes and infant care classes may be offered virtually, at your hospital, in your home, or in a birth center, and are taught by trained childbirth educators. Some are specific to home birth, unmedicated birth, or use specific pain-relief methods such as visualization.
- **Prenatal fitness or yoga classes:** Many virtual or in-person offerings for prenatal yoga, Pilates, cardio, and other classes are available. Seek guidance from your pelvic physical therapist or physician before signing up.
- **Prenatal dietician or nutrition expert:** Seek out registered dieticians or licensed nutritionists who are specifically trained to focus on optimized prenatal nutrition for both growth and wellness of you and your baby and can help you to manage gestational diabetes or navigate other health issues during pregnancy.
- **Breathwork coach:** A breathwork coach can train you to use your breath for mindfulness, relaxation, and pain management.
- **Reiki practitioner:** Reiki is a form of energy healing that promotes wellness and relaxation among other benefits and is performed lightly hands-on while you remain fully clothed.
- **Prenatal massage practitioner:** Massage therapists can help you connect to your changing body, relax, relieve aches and pains, and assist with swelling. Look for one that has specific prenatal training.

- **Craniosacral therapist:** A gentle hands-on approach to body healing and releasing of tensions, craniosacral therapy is relaxing and is performed while you are fully clothed.
- **Acupuncturist:** An acupuncturist is trained in a form of Traditional Chinese Medicine that uses fine needles to target energy meridians in the body for healing and well-being. Acupuncture can also help prepare your body to go into labor in the final weeks/days of pregnancy.
- **Mental health therapist:** There are therapists who specialize specifically in working with pregnant or postpartum people and/or their partners. Look for a licensed therapist, which includes clinical social workers to doctors of psychology.
- **Support groups:** There are so many offerings that I love, whether in person or virtual, that provide new parents and caregivers with breastfeeding, parenthood, or other birthing or postpartum support. These groups are opportunities for support as well as community, which is especially helpful in the sometimes-isolating time immediately postpartum.

A Word on Mental Health: Birth is a Big Deal

I would be remiss if I did not address mental health postpartum. Such extensive preparation goes toward labor and delivery and making so many tiny yet major choices for early parenthood— and it can feel like once Baby arrives, all focus is placed on the new little person. But both the act of birth and the transition to parenthood can be a lot to cope with. It could be that you need some help processing a birth that didn't go as planned, dealing with sleep deprivation, and/or navigating the onset of major life changes, in addition to anxiety, depression, fear—or a multitude of other reasons. Whatever the case may be, I encourage you to speak to your midwife, OB/GYN, or a member of your care team and find a licensed mental health professional who can hear you out—and offer help.

And now, onto the goods.

Dr. Sam's Exercise Essentials

Through many years of seeing clients and hands-on experience building and directing pelvic physical therapy clinics, I've put together this carefully curated list of workout accessories and equipment that will safely elevate your exercise routine. Note that none of these are must-haves, just "nice-to-haves" if you're in the market.

Workout Gear

ITEM	NOTES
Yoga Mat	When it comes to yoga mats, I recommend eco-friendly ones that are made of sustainable material and without the toxic chemicals typically used to soften rubber. Get yourself one with at least 6mm thickness—it will give your knees, hands, and wrists extra cushioning love during pregnancy. Bonus: great for baby or toddler yoga in the future!
Hand Weights	A versatile set of weights allows you to perform and modify a range of exercises right at home—including upper body, lower body and core. No need to spend much here; just snag a set in a weight range that's right for you. I like a pair of 5, 8, and 10-lb weights for the average person.
Kettlebell	Great for adding low-grade weight to a squat, a kettlebell makes a smart alternative or addition to your weight set. See a pelvic physical therapist (either in-person or virtually) to learn how to control your intra-abdominal pressure if you plan to perform kettlebell swings or other dynamic movements. I like the coated ones for easier gripping.
Resistance Bands	A set of strong, stretchy bands offer another easy way to take your workout on-the-go, whether you're traveling or just squeezing in some reps between meetings. You can perform upper body and lower body exercises with these bands, adding resistance to almost any exercise, like bridges, lunges, squats, and side-stepping.
Bolster Pillow	Restorative yoga and stretching are great for a tired, growing body. Settle in and get comfortable with the help of a posture-perfecting bolster pillow. Use it to help melt into a stretch, practice breathwork, or meditate. Bonus: Use this pillow as a bolster in bed for propping up during late-night feeding sessions postpartum or practicing tummy time with baby.

Workout Apparel

ITEM	NOTES
Workout One-Piece	A workout onesie is easy to slip on and off, whether you're in the prenatal stage or lactating postpartum, and a crossed back is ideal for supporting your growing breast tissue. Look for one that's buttery soft—perfect for pregnancy—and breathable during those extra hot flashes.
Sports Bra	Find yourself a great sports bra with wide shoulder straps to support your posture. Your breast size and shape will change throughout pregnancy and postpartum, so you may need several options. Look for a supportive bra that does not overly compress the breast tissue, especially if you intend to lactate, pump, or breastfeed, as tight compression can lead to painful clogged ducts. Many retailers now do custom fittings and will add hooks on the front straps to convert any bra into a nursing bra.
Compression Socks	Compression socks provide light support for swollen feet and ankles, especially when you can't put your legs up the wall between clients, work meetings, or simply parenting. Reminder: Swelling in your vulvar area, ankles, feet, and legs should always be checked out by your doctor if you have pitting (when you push your finger in and the dent stays), if it is painful, or if it is sudden in onset. If you have a cardiac or wound-healing condition, also ask your medical provider first before using compression socks.

Belly band? It's complicated.

One of the most common questions I get is about belly support bands. Belly bands won't give you enough support if you're showing signs of tenting, doming, bulging, or other symptoms of DR or if you're carrying very low or having pain.

In those cases, I'd prescribe specific support garments to facilitate your abdominal muscles, in addition to changing your movements, modifying your breath, and person-to-person specific techniques and exercises.

Otherwise, readily available belly bands or even high-waisted leggings are all most people will need for a small amount of added support and comfort during pregnancy. Choose something that's comfortable, washes easily, and is breathable, especially on those hot days.

Postpartum? Toss the bands. Unless belly banding (or abdominal wrapping) is a traditional part of your culture—in which case, make sure it is loose enough that you can easily tuck two fingers into the bands. All that extra pressure tightly around the abdomen can put pressure downward on the pelvic floor organs—and we want to keep those right where they are.

CHAPTER 10:

Setting Expectations

You've had your baby—now what?

The twelve-week timeframe postpartum is often referred to as the fourth trimester, due to its great physical and emotional transformation. It varies from person to person in terms of the immediate postpartum experience, especially in terms of the kind of labor and delivery you had. First and foremost, the focus is on your immediate health and your baby's. This also includes learning how to feed your baby, whether that is by breastfeeding, a breast pump, or bottle-feeding. How you nourish your baby is a very personal decision and there is no universal "right" way—just like there is no one right way to conceive or birth a baby. If you choose to go the route of breastfeeding, lactation support is often a crucial resource for many. I strongly encourage utilizing help with latch, feeding, understanding length and timing of feeds, and so forth.

The first few weeks, the baby is often on a two-hour schedule: wake, eat, diaper change, sleep (or some semblance of this.) You are adjusting to caring for a new, helpless human; dealing with sleep deprivation; and caring for yourself and possibly other children. Be gentle on yourself and your expectations.

The first few days postpartum, you will likely experience swelling, some loss in sensation around the area of a surgical site/scar (if you had a c-section birth), discharge, bleeding, and potentially some incontinence or pain. The good news is you've put together a postpartum dream team, who is there to help you with these things, from ice packs to pain moderation, to helping you get stool moving for your first (often uncomfortable) bowel movement postpartum. My best advice to you during the first few days: DON'T PANIC! How you look and feel the first days will change dramatically and quickly.

After discharge from immediate care as advised by your birth provider, your care team will advise you of certain things to look out for that may warrant a call back to them. These might include an increase in pain, bleeding, full bladder loss, full fecal incontinence, and so forth. Heed their advice and advocate for yourself: by now, you are intimately connected with your body and its cues. If something doesn't feel right, ask a medical professional.

Your primary goals in the first 30 days postpartum are nourishment, readjustment, utilization of resources, finding a new routine, and caring for yourself and your baby. While you are recovering, be gracious and patient with your body. Listen closely to its cues and take it one day (or one hour) at a time.

If you have a partner, you may want to consider exploring and learning together about what your partnership will look like around the time of delivery, what resources you'd most benefit from immediately, and over the first 3-6 months postpartum. Sharing this book with your partner may even be a good idea.

Your Body

Many people feel like the goal is to get back to a pre-pregnancy body, routine, and life, but physically this isn't entirely possible for all bodies. Your body just underwent the **greatest** physical transformation possible in human life. You might find that some of the things you did before giving birth just may not be possible— at least right now. And giving up the things you love to do, the exhaustion, the physical and mental transformation— all of it can be a really difficult thing to manage.

As a runner, I was hit hard when I realized I couldn't start running again right away. I love to run. I love the autonomy, the meditative quality, and it's how I feel most free. It also provides me with an emotional and mental release. Yet I could not run for quite some time postpartum. Again, I encourage you to be gentle with yourself and give yourself some grace to explore new outlets for emotional or physical release, at least until your body is in a place to resume your usual activities.

It will take approximately 4-6 weeks for the lochia (postpartum bleeding) to cease and for your uterus to return to its original size and position in the body. During this time, work on deep breathing, finding that gentle connection to your body. At about 12-14 days postpartum, begin gentle transverse abdominal contractions (if you have not had a c-section) and take slow, short walks. The hormones that supported your pregnancy are rapidly leaving your body, which may cause effects like hot flashes and sweats. Foot swelling will go down, and your shoe size might even change slightly. Use a small hand mirror and take a peek at your vulvar area and notice any changes.

Most people see their OB/GYN or midwife at 4-6 weeks postpartum for "clearance" to exercise or have sex. This is also a great time to see your pelvic physical therapist to discuss progression to next steps, your goals, and physical recovery.

Finally, you might feel less familiar or connected to your pregnant or postpartum body—and that's normal. Not everyone loves breastfeeding, or a softer belly, and some find it hard to honor the stretch marks or scars. That is also okay. Be intentional as you go through the exercises and practices of this book. Pay attention to the movement of the body and how all things are connected, working together in constant communication. It's incredible.

This is your body and carrying a child—then caring for a new life—is a major deal. You did this. You! Your magnificent body! Congratulations!

CLOSING

Wishing you a confident, safe, and beautiful birth.

Throughout your pregnancy, your health and the health of your baby are the most important things. You now have many of the resources—make the time to support yourself! If you don't feel like you're loving pregnancy, you're not alone— getting through it takes more work for some of us than others.

Do the work. You will never regret the decision to feel as good as you can. Knowledge is power, friends, and I hope this information helps you feel confident and in control of your body. Supporting yourself and your physical well-being is a great step in self-advocacy during pregnancy, and a true form of self-care. Keep trusting in your one and only body.

Deep breath—you got this!

Dr. Sam

ABOUT DR. SAM

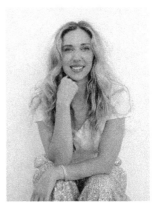

D r. Sam DuFlo, PT, DPT, PRPC is a nationally known and acclaimed physical therapist and leader in pelvic floor health, and the founder and Chief Medical Officer of Indigo Physiotherapy. Through her clinical practice, work as adjunct faculty at a number of universities, and medical outreach and research, Dr. Sam is driving a new paradigm of care.

When Dr. Sam gave birth to her child in 2018—gaining firsthand knowledge of the joys of pregnancy, from epic morning sickness to pelvic congestion, to birthing a sunny-side up (or direct occiput posterior [OP]) baby—her journey through pregnancy and birth led her to search for better answers and guidance. And that void was all the reason she needed to create an easy, accessible resource for parents who want to prepare for their most empowered and physically capable birth.

In her day-to-day work, she uses and teaches an integrated approach, incorporating therapeutic and manual techniques to help clients navigate pregnancy, birth, postpartum recovery, menstrual changes, pelvic pain and dysfunction, and sexual health. Recognizing the gap in the traditional health care system for birthing persons, Dr. Sam's work centers on treating and strengthening the whole pregnant person. Ultimately, she strives to lead clients to achieve their birthing goals and have easier birth recoveries.

ABOUT INDIGO PHYSIOTHERAPY

Founded by Dr. Sam DuFlo in 2016, Indigo Physiotherapy challenges the traditional models of care by offering a more individualized, comprehensive level of pelvic and orthopedic physical therapy that elevates the client experience and empowers patients through education and advocacy.

After suffering a running injury in her 30's and going through recovery, Dr. Sam went back to school to become a doctor of physical therapy. As one of the older students in the class with more life experience, she found she also had more questions. Why should doctors camouflage their character under khaki and polos? Why should treatment rooms be stripped of comfort and warmth? And why all the red tape and regulation from the insurance powers that be?

From these questions and voids grew the vision for Indigo. Today, Indigo is the largest and leading pelvic floor physical therapy practice in the U.S., and continues to exclusively offer one-on-one, personalized pelvic physical therapy and bodywork treatment, focused on individual goals for healing and function.

REFERENCES

Abdelhakim, A. M., Eldesouky, E., Elmagd, I. A., Mohammed, A., Farag, E. A., Mohammed, A. E., Hamam, K. M., Hussein, A. S., Ali, A. S., Keshta, N. H. A., Hamza, M., Samy, A., & Abdel-Latif, A. A. (2020). Antenatal perineal massage benefits in reducing perineal trauma and postpartum morbidities: a systematic review and meta-analysis of randomized controlled trials. International Urogynecology Journal. https://doi.org/10.1007/s00192-020-04302-8

ACOG Practice Bulletin No. 198. (2018). Obstetrics & Gynecology, 132(3), e87–e102. https://doi.org/10.1097/aog.0000000000002841

Alex, A., Bhandary, E., & McGuire, K. P. (2020). Anatomy and Physiology of the Breast during Pregnancy and Lactation. Advances in Experimental Medicine and Biology, 1252, 3–7. https://doi.org/10.1007/978-3-030-41596-9_1

Aquino, C. I., Guida, M., Saccone, G., Cruz, Y., Vitagliano, A., Zullo, F., & Berghella, V. (2018). Perineal massage during labor: a systematic review and meta-analysis of randomized controlled trials. The Journal of Maternal-Fetal & Neonatal Medicine, 33(6), 1051–1063. https://doi.org/10.1080/14767058.2018.1512574

Barakat, R., Pelaez, M., Lopez, C., Montejo, R., & Coteron, J. (2012). Exercise during pregnancy reduces the rate of cesarean and instrumental deliveries: results of a randomized controlled trial. The Journal of Maternal-Fetal & Neonatal Medicine, 25(11), 2372–2376. https://doi.org/10.3109/14767058.2012.696165

Beckmann, M. M., & Stock, O. M. (2013). Antenatal perineal massage for reducing perineal trauma. Cochrane Database of Systematic Reviews, 4. https://doi.org/10.1002/14651858.cd005123.pub3

Blomquist, J. L., Carroll, M., Muñoz, A., & Handa, V. L. (2020). Pelvic floor muscle strength and the incidence of pelvic floor disorders after vaginal and cesarean delivery. American Journal of Obstetrics and Gynecology, 222(1), 62.e1–62.e8. https://doi.org/10.1016/j.ajog.2019.08.003

Body, C., & Christie, J. A. (2016). Gastrointestinal Diseases in Pregnancy. Gastroenterology Clinics of North America, 45(2), 267–283. https://doi.org/10.1016/j.gtc.2016.02.005

Cao, X., Yang, Q., Wang, Q., Hu, S., Hou, L., Sun, M., Lai, H., Wu, C., Wu, Y., Xiao, L., Luo, X., Tian, J., Ge, L., & Luo, C. (2022). PFMT relevant strategies to prevent perineal trauma: a systematic review and network meta-analysis. Archives of Gynecology and Obstetrics. https://doi.org/10.1007/s00404-022-06769-w

Cavalli, M., Aiolfi, A., Bruni, P. G., Manfredini, L., Lombardo, F., Bonfanti, M. T., Bona, D., & Campanelli, G. (2021). Prevalence and risk factors for diastasis recti abdominis: a review and proposal of a new anatomical variation. Hernia, 25(4), 883–890. https://doi.org/10.1007/s10029-021-02468-8

Chiou, W.-K., Chiu, H.-T., Chao, A.-S., Wang, M.-H., & Chen, Y.-L. (2015). The influence of body mass on foot dimensions during pregnancy. Applied Ergonomics, 46, 212–217. https://doi. org/10.1016/j.apergo.2014.08.004

Cho, S. T., & Kim, K. H. (2021). Pelvic floor muscle exercise and training for coping with urinary incontinence. Journal of Exercise Rehabilitation, 17(6), 379–387. https://doi.org/10.12965/ jer.2142666.333

Connolly, C. P., Conger, S. A., Montoye, A. H. K., Marshall, M. R., Schlaff, R. A., Badon, S. E., & Pivarnik, J. M. (2018). Walking for health during pregnancy: A literature review and considerations for future research. Journal of Sport and Health Science, 8(5). https://doi.org/10.1016/j.jshs.2018.11.004

Davari Tanha, F., Ghajarzadeh, M., Mohseni, M., Shariat, M., & Ranjbar, M. (2014). Is ACOG guideline helpful for encouraging pregnant women to do exercise during pregnancy? Acta Medica Iranica, 52(6), 458–461. https://www.ncbi.nlm.nih.gov/ pubmed/25130154

Davenport, M. H. (2020). EXERCISE DURING PREGNANCY: A Prescription for Improved Maternal/Fetal Well-being. ACSM'S Health & Fitness Journal, 24(5), 10–17. https://doi.org/10.1249/ fit.0000000000000602

Dieb, A. S., Shoab, A. Y., Nabil, H., Gabr, A., Abdallah, A. A., Shaban, M. M., & Attia, A. H. (2019). Perineal massage and training reduce perineal trauma in pregnant women older than 35 years: a randomized controlled trial. International Urogynecology Journal. https://doi.org/10.1007/s00192-019-03937-6

Dunn, J., Dunn, C., Habbu, R., Bohay, D., & Anderson, J. (2012). Effect of Pregnancy and Obesity on Arch of Foot. Orthopaedic Surgery, 4(2), 101–104. https://doi.org/10.1111/j.1757-7861.2012.00179.x Exercise During Pregnancy. (2019, July). www.acog.org. https://www.acog.org/womens-health/faqs/exercise-during-pregnancy

Freeman, M. E., Kanyicska, B., Lerant, A., & Nagy, G. (2000). Prolactin: structure, function, and regulation of secretion. Physiological Reviews, 80(4), 1523–1631. https://doi.org/10.1152/physrev.2000.80.4.1523

Gluppe, S., Engh, M. E., & Bø, K. (2021). What is the evidence for abdominal and pelvic floor muscle training to treat diastasis recti abdominis postpartum? A systematic review with meta-analysis. Brazilian Journal of Physical Therapy, 25(6). https://doi.org/10.1016/j.bjpt.2021.06.006

Gomes, C. F., Sousa, M., Lourenço, I., Martins, D., & Torres, J. (2018). Gastrointestinal diseases during pregnancy: what does the gastroenterologist need to know? Annals of Gastroenterology, 31(4), 385–394. https://doi.org/10.20524/aog.2018.0264

Grattan, D. R., & Ladyman, S. R. (2020). Neurophysiological and cognitive changes in pregnancy. Handbook of Clinical Neurology, 171, 25–55. https://doi.org/10.1016/B978-0-444-64239-4.00002-3

Huang, Y.-C., & Chang, K.-V. (2021). Kegel Exercises. PubMed; StatPearls Publishing. https://www.ncbi.nlm.nih.gov/books/ NBK555898/

Igualada-Martinez, P. (2020, February 20). 50 years of Physiotherapy. ICS. https://www.ics.org/news/1047

Lawson, S., & Sacks, A. (2018). Pelvic Floor Physical Therapy and Women's Health Promotion. Journal of Midwifery & Women's Health, 63(4), 410–417. https://doi.org/10.1111/jmwh.12736

Leon-Larios, F., Corrales-Gutierrez, I., Casado-Mejía, R., & Suarez-Serrano, C. (2017). Influence of a pelvic floor training programme to prevent perineal trauma: A quasi-randomised controlled trial. Midwifery, 50, 72–77. https://doi.org/10.1016/j. midw.2017.03.015

Maternity and Post-Operative Exercises in Diagrams and Words. (1937). Journal of the American Medical Association, 108(25), 2161. https://doi.org/10.1001/jama.1937.02780250075028

Melzer, K., Schutz, Y., Boulvain, M., & Kayser, B. (2010). Physical Activity and Pregnancy. Sports Medicine, 40(6), 493–507. https:// doi.org/10.2165/11532290-000000000-00000

Padayachee, C. (2015). Exercise guidelines for gestational diabetes mellitus. World Journal of Diabetes, 6(8), 1033. https://doi. org/10.4239/wjd.v6.i8.1033

Page, P. (2012). Current concepts in muscle stretching for exercise and rehabilitation. International Journal of Sports Physical Therapy, 7(1), 109–119. https://pubmed.ncbi.nlm.nih.gov/22319684/

Rana, M., Jain, S., & Choubey, P. (2022). Prolactin and its significance in the placenta. Hormones, 21(2), 209–219. https://doi.org/10.1007/s42000-022-00373-y

Serna-Hoyos, L. C., Herrón Arango, A. F., Ortiz-Mesa, S., Vieira-Rios, S. M., Arbelaez-Lelion, D., Vanegas-Munera, J. M., & Castillo-Bustamante, M. (2022). Vertigo in Pregnancy: A Narrative Review. Cureus, 14(5). https://doi.org/10.7759/cureus.25386

Ugwu, E. O., Iferikigwe, E. S., Obi, S. N., Eleje, G. U., & Ozumba, B. C. (2018). Effectiveness of antenatal perineal massage in reducing perineal trauma and post-partum morbidities: A randomized controlled trial. Journal of Obstetrics and Gynaecology Research, 44(7), 1252–1258. https://doi.org/10.1111/jog.13640

Vargas-Terrones, M., Nagpal, T. S., & Barakat, R. (2019). Impact of exercise during pregnancy on gestational weight gain and birth weight: an overview. Brazilian Journal of Physical Therapy, 23(2), 164–169. https://doi.org/10.1016/j.bjpt.2018.11.012

Wang, Y. H. W., & Wiseman, J. (2022). Anatomy, Abdomen and Pelvis, Rectum. PubMed; StatPearls Publishing. https://www.ncbi.nlm.nih.gov/pubmed/30725930

World Health Organization. (2022, October 5). Physical activity. Physical Activity; World Health Organization. https://www.who.int/news-room/fact-sheets/detail/physical-activity

World Health Organization. (2012). Use and procurement of additional lubricants for male and female condoms: WHO/ UNFPA/FHI360: advisory note. Apps.who.int. https://apps.who. int/iris/handle/10665/76580

A free ebook edition is available with the purchase of this book.

To claim your free ebook edition:
1. Visit MorganJamesBOGO.com
2. Sign your name CLEARLY in the space
3. Complete the form and submit a photo of the entire copyright page
4. You or your friend can download the ebook to your preferred device

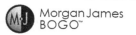

Morgan James
BOGO™

A **FREE** ebook edition is available for you or a friend with the purchase of this print book.

CLEARLY SIGN YOUR NAME ABOVE

Instructions to claim your free ebook edition:
1. Visit MorganJamesBOGO.com
2. Sign your name CLEARLY in the space above
3. Complete the form and submit a photo of this entire page
4. You or your friend can download the ebook to your preferred device

Print & Digital Together Forever.

Snap a photo   Free ebook   Read anywhere

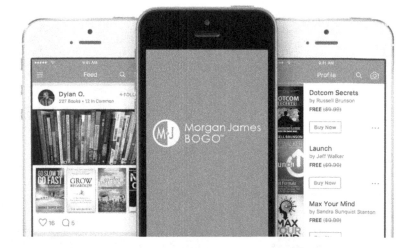

Printed in the USA
CPSIA information can be obtained
at www.ICGtesting.com
JSHW080319111123
51877JS00002B/6